IT'S ME, I'VE COME

ALSO BY THE SAME AUTHOR
Threads of Circumstance

In Preparation
What is Life Without Adventure

IT'S ME, I'VE COME

by

Ruby Dymond

Regency Press (London & New York) Ltd.
125 High Holborn, London WC1V 6QA

First Published 1985
New Edition 1994

To my friend
John Thorpe

ISBN 0 7212 0834 7

Printed and bound in Great Britain by
Buckland Press Ltd., Dover, Kent.

CONTENTS

	Page
Chapter One	7
Chapter Two	12
Chapter Three	17
Chapter Four	25
Chapter Five	32
Chapter Six	36
Chapter Seven	43
Chapter Eight	51
Chapter Nine	59
Chapter Ten	68
Chapter Eleven	74
Chapter Twelve	80
Chapter Thirteen	94
Chapter Fourteen	100
Chapter Fifteen	104
Chapter Sixteen	111
Chapter Seventeen	124
Chapter Eighteen	132
Chapter Nineteen	141
Chapter Twenty	147

LIST OF ILLUSTRATIONS

	Page
Sister 'Dolly' Thistlethwayte	81
St. Mary's Hospital	81
The Matron of St. Mary's surrounded by a group of her Sisters	82
Nurses receiving a lesson in the Preliminary Training School, prior to their actual work in the wards	82
Ruby Morris in St. Mary's Theatre	83
Sister with a new school of probationers	83
Nurse M. J. Gatward, charge nurse, the maternity ward in 1931	84
Sister in the maternity ward, 1930	84
The author in Foochow, 1938, at the Kushan Monastery	85
A painting on silk by Dr. Dymond, the author's husband	85
E. C. Dymond, aged 20	86
The author, aged 35, taken in Shanghai	86
Nurse Irene Drake	87
Bill Peacock, Irene Drake and Ruby Morris, 1926	87
Husky and Ruby, 1926	88
Jimmy Dymond and Nurse Huskinson	88

Chapter One

"When I grow up I'm going to travel and travel! But I'll never be a nurse, I'll never marry a doctor; and I shall *never* go to China." "Now, Ruby," warned my gentle mother, "you must *not* be so emphatic, or you will surely do all three."

From as early as I can remember, the words acting, theatre, and cinema, had held a magic for me, and during my adolescence, in the early 'twenties, my ambitions flared to white heat. This, in spite of my father's fond boast that, "Dear little Ruby – such a contented child," had never brought him a day's trouble in his life.

No one, not even my brother George, suspected the intense life of poetry and drama that went on in my imagination. Outwardly, I was a calm, quiet child and when missing, could usually be found in some secluded corner of the garden, deep in a volume of Shakespeare, Dickens, or fairy-tales.

Father's business firm transferred him from town to town, so our family was constantly being uprooted. And as soon as we were once more settled, Father searched for a suitable chapel and every Sunday we'd sally forth, Father in frock-coat and silk hat, a flower in his lapel, Mother looking adorable in her latest chic hat, and we three children in our best Sunday clothes. Having tried every denomination, Father settled for the minister with the most fiery delivery. Great was his happiness when he found a Welsh minister with the gift of the 'hwyl'.

The first thing I did was to find the local cemetery in which I felt perfectly happy and at ease. These faithful searchings and absences of mine became the butt of a family joke. A typical answer to the query, "Where's Ruby?" was, "Oh, she's either at the bottom of the garden reading, in the cemetery, or gazing at the moon."

Father was an ardent upholder of chapel-going, and with his fine tenor voice, was an inspiring choir-master. He was happy too at the discovery that I had an unusually powerful voice, and from an early age, a true ear for pitch. As time went on he trained my voice, and often made me the soloist in his choirs.

Listeners, they say, never hear any good of themselves. I remember when very young, listening at the drawing-room door wherein Mother was entertaining a friend to tea, and clearly came mother's anxious voice:

"Oh, Olwen fach, I'm worried."

"Worried, dear, what about?"

"It's that child, Ruby, forever with her head in a book; always plaguing us for books, books, books!"

"No harm surely in books, is there, dear?" soothed Olwen.

"In themselves, no. But it's her imagination; always talking to her 'people' as she calls them. Every night when she's in bed, George and I listen to her, he thinks it's not healthy, Olwen."

"Well," replied Olwen firmly, "I'm absolutely *sure* that child will end up on the stage."

A small gasp of horror came from Mother.

"On the stage! Oh, Olwen, fach, I'd rather see little Ruby dead, and in her grave . . . On the *stage* . . . No child of mine will *ever* go on the stage . . ."

I crept away passionately hugging to myself my great secret; the joyous dream of being a famous dramatic actress. Passionate, too, was my adoration of those whom I considered God-like people; bitter indeed were my feelings when these idols fell from their pedestals. However, such was my devotion that invariably I'd find an excuse to pop them back again. And so, from the age of six my mind floated on a cloud of fantastic imagination. My bedroom at night was peopled by a variety of imaginary characters, whom I entertained with animated conversation. I was never alone, for my 'people' came with me everywhere.

Brother George, three years older than myself was also an idealistic temperament. Throughout childhood, George was my hero and constant companion. Together we fell passionately in love, he with the Gish sisters, and I with the then world's sweetheart, Mary Pickford. Every night found us ardently praying for their welfare. One day I remember when deep in a book, I was jerked out of its pages when Father came home and boomed out to my Mother:

"*Another* film star in the divorce court, Jinnie!" he flung his newspaper down on the table.

I felt as though a knife plunged into my heart for I *knew* he was going to say, "Mary Pickford, of all people!" I marched out of the room, up the stairs and into my bedroom, and flung myself down on the bed and sobbed with unspeakable grief. Nothing consoled me, neither would I say what was the matter; I remember Father saying anxiously to Mother; "Jinnie, this child is sick". Then on a sudden inspiration he touched me gently: "Ruby, are you crying about Mary Pickford?"

I nodded dumbly:

"But, Ruby bach, you foolish little girl," he said quite seriously, "It's not *Mary* who's been naughty – it's her husband."

I'd no idea at all of the significance of the 'naughty' but my sobs ceased and in no time at all Mary was back on her pedestal. All through those early years I went on falling dramatically in and out of love, in and out of love. The objects of my passion seldom knew the enchantment they cast over me – I was content to worship from afar. And instead of touching, I communed with the moon, stars and all things fair in nature, it seemed to me they would understand.

A crisis came into mine and George's life on the day when cinema placards announced that a Mary Pickford, William Farnum and Lilian Gish film was to be shown in the *same week.* The placard stated, 'Coming Shortly'. This was sheer tragedy, for our loyalties could not be divided. We were seldom allowed to go to the cinema, and never alone.

The next day when we were rummaging in the attic, George came across a small cardboard box in which was a set of old false teeth. (We never did discover to whom they belonged.) George gazed at them with rapt attention – I with nausea. A few moments and he came out of his reverie and whispered excitedly; "Three pictures in one week – we need three shillings! Rubes," he went on using his pet name for me, "Rubes, we can *sell* these teeth. I've seen a shop that says they buy them!"

"Dare we, George," I whispered back, anxious yet hopeful, "Isn't it stealing?"

"Don't be silly," said my brother, impatiently, "of course it isn't, *we* found them and anyway, Dad and Mummy haven't got false teeth, so it can't be stealing, can it?"

Cautiously we crept down the stairs and out of the house. Filled with the spirit of adventure we stepped smartly into town. George entered the shop alone and when he emerged a few minutes later, he was quivering with excitement. Slowly, he opened his hand – there lay seven whole shillings and sixpence!

Thus, for the first time in our young lives, and due to our devotion to three film stars, we were led into the path of deception; and during the 'big week' when Mother fondly believed us to be playing in the park, there we were sitting in the sixpennies, holding hands in a state of ecstatic expectation, while the lady in a black dress and bun, pounded from the piano what to us seemed wildly exciting music.

We came home floating on rosy clouds.

But gradually, our triumph turned to gall, for our consciences were troubled. At Sunday School, from a prominent position on a wall, a gilt-edged text stated; "Thou God Seest All" and the eye painted above it pierced our hearts.

Shortly after our submitting to temptation, two famous evangelists, Mr. Fred, and Arthur Wood, came to Southport and held revival meetings in the Town Hall. We were attracted by the long white banner with its scarlet letters announcing; 'Young Life Campaigners – All Welcome'. A wave of religious fervour swept like a fire through the town, and we were swept along with it. We attended the meetings with heavily laden consciences, sitting inconspicuously at the back of the hall – two small, overwhelmed children. In hypnotic trance, we watched the grown-ups responding to the urgent summons: "Come up and be saved! Come up and be saved! Don't wait, friends, don't wait – come right up and be saved."

We were the last in the slowly moving line that wended its way towards the back room – and salvation. When our turn came the ardent young men escorted us inside; no hint of amusement crept into their eyes when we knelt down and bleated out fervently:

"We have sinned!"

George poured forth the sad story of the false teeth, the subsequent lies and the three unauthorised visits to the cinema. By the end of the painful but exhilarating interview, we were well and truly saved. We solemnly signed the pledge, which bound us for evermore to abstain from alcoholic drink, and we faithfully promised never to deceive our parents again.

As we made our way home through the golden sunset, George was unusually quiet. Suddenly he stopped and said despairingly; "Rubes, I *cannot* give up Lilian Gish!"

And I replied in anguish, "Oh, dear, and I can't give up Mary and William."

There were still a few sixpences left, and after a serious discussion we settled for a compromise – we'd remain faithful to our loves and if forced to tell more lies to see them, we'd pray for forgiveness. And we prayed harder than ever for our idols.

Our other great love, a love who had no rival, was our Old English sheep dog, Rossie. She and I came into the family at the same time and we grew up together. No matter where we three children went Rossie would follow. She knew she was our guardian. Every summer at the first signs of packing she would share our transport of delight – packing to go down into Wales!

Wales! The land of magic and wonder.

The most enchanted days of our childhood were spent at our grandparents' farm, 'Hendre Mawr', near the village of Llanuwchllyn, where Father was born. We called our grandparents 'Taid' and 'Nain' in the Welsh way. Mother too was Welsh, she was born in Barmouth, and we could never decide which of the two places was the more enchanting. Taid was a tall old gentleman with wrinkled cheeks and gnarled hands. He had a drooping white moustache, and a merry twinkle in his deep blue eyes. Nain was a jolly, fat little lady, energetic and practical. She it was who ran the farm, successfully too, for Taid was a dreamer and a poet. I felt very close to him. What awe when allowed to sit in the old bardic chair in which he'd been crowned at the Eisteddfod, I would sit there as long as possible, basking in reflected glory.

Often he hoisted me onto his shoulder, and instead of obeying orders to go and mend hedges, the pair of us would sneak off, and escape to the top of the huge haystack. I clearly recall the sweet, clean smell of the hay as, curled up in the crook of his arm, I shared his silences. And stared up into the blue dome of the sky, watching the white, woolly clouds racing across the heavens. Sometimes Taid would be taken with the 'hwyl' and in his rich voice start reciting his own poems in Welsh. The musical cadences in his voice filled me with a vague sorrow, and made me weep with a sadness I didn't understand:

"It's nice, Ruby fach," he whispered, on one of these occasions, "nice indeed that you understand my poetry without knowing the Welsh but it's sad I am that your Tada hasn't taught you," he looked down at me and went on dreamily, "All the same, fach, you're ver-ry Welsh. Did you know that your grandtaid sang like an angel? Ninety-two he was when he died. Yes, indeed, he actually died while singing 'Jesu, Lover of my Soul' to the Aberystwyth tune – beau-ti-ful it was. It's his gift that you've inherited, so sing, fach, sing."

There was no escape from singing in that little chapel below the farm. Every Sunday the minister would ask me to sing some hymns after the sermon. And when at last the congregation rose to sing the last hymn, Nain, in her old, but penetrating voice, led them to repeat the last verse. Over and over again the challenge of, "Bread of Heaven, feed me now and evermore . . ." rose in such intense crescendo of emotion I trembled for fear the very building would collapse.

And so the years rolled by, and I lived in a world totally divorced from reality. At school, which, of necessity changed with each family uprooting, I received praise for only three subjects – essay-writing, singing and reciting poetry. All the various teachers thought me a studious child – until it was discovered that my quiet concentration was on fairy-tales, surreptitiously placed between the leaves of history and geography books.

Chapter Two

Sorrow came slyly into our lives when Mother, at forty, became pregnant. The disturbing secret was revealed only to our sister, Cassie, who adored Mother, and was always the closest to her. George and I knew nothing about the new baby until the very last minute, when we were packed off for the day to a neighbour, and when we got back, Father said:

"Go upstairs now, and see your new sister."

We shyly kissed Mother, then stared down at the fragile bundle in the cradle. We had stopped asking the 'where do babies come from' questions, being unsatisfied with stock Victorian answers of storks and fairies. The mystery remained but the baby we accepted with joy. Rossie, who'd followed us up the stairs, was bitterly hurt at this intrusion of this rival for our affections. On hearing the exclamations of delight, down went her bobtail, she looked up at us reproachfully and crept away under Mother's bed.

In the heedless way of children, all our attention was now centred on the baby, who was christened Eirlys Olwen, but whom we nick-named Lilas. Although Rossie showed no animosity towards her tiny rival, she quietly grieved herself to death, and then too late, we children were broken-hearted. It seemed an ill omen too, for Mother never completely recovered her strength, and soon developed tuberculosis.

When the doctor told Father nothing could save the life of the wife with whom he'd lived in the closest harmony for twenty-five years, he was inconsolable. I cannot recall ever hearing our parents quarrelling nor do I remember ever seeing Mother angry – always, she was a gentle, kind and considerate person.

The disease progressed slowly and when she became bedridden, my school-days had ended – I was barely fourteen. The delicate baby became my sole charge, while Cassie, with great devotion nursed Mother until her death, two years later of meningitis.

This was my first encounter with death. I went into the bedroom alone; although my heart was thumping wildly I was not afraid. She lay between snowy sheets – a frail, marble angel – and in her slender fingers was a bunch of Lilies of the Valley. Their fragrance filled the room; I stood still with tightly closed eyes – it seemed to me the room was filled too with softly fluttering wings . . .

It was spring when Cassie got married and went to live in Llanuwchllyn; thereafter, with the aid of cook-housemaids who came and went with the frequency of April showers, I took charge of our home. Since leaving school, my passion for acting had deepened. Lilas was quite used to hearing me rendering impassioned speeches, tenderly recited poems and sad Celtic songs, in which I indulged while pushing her about in her pram. This dearly loved little sister was very like her mother, her eyes held the same appealing doe-like expression. Neighbours, seeing how delicate she looked would prophesy in my hearing "Jinnie Morris's child will never grow up."

This remark worried me into sleepless nights, I lay awake for hours listening to her breathing and at times when I couldn't hear it, my heart raced with terror. During that time Father and George were often away from home. My brother had joined Father's firm and was travelling all over the country. My white-hot ambition, to become a dramatic actress was unshaken; hours I spent in front of a mirror, studying expressions and making up into various characters. One vivid character I remember to this day. The impersonation was of 'Madame X', a character from a film I'd seen in which the only thing I understood was that the poor lady was drinking herself to death with absinthe.

One evening, on the cook's night off, and I was alone in the house with Lilas, a heavy, dramatic mood overcame me. After settling my sister in bed, I solemnly gathered materials to transform myself into the role of Madame X; flour, a burnt cork, eye-brush, tumbler and jug of water, mirror and an old shawl. These I placed reverently on the kitchen table and drew up a chair.

The procedure of turning the pale, chubby face before me into that of the desperate woman took a considerable time. With whitened hair and a couple of blacked out teeth I went on with the makeup, the while sipping the water which had now turned into the lethal absinthe; under its influence the tragic brown eyes darkened. The face staring at me from the mirror was truly ghastly – great hollow eyes, wispy hair and shawl around cringing shoulders.

Deep and deeper I sank into the state of suicidal drunkenness; then – just as I'd reached the stage of heart-broken sobs – the door suddenly opened, and I lifted my ravaged face to my brother George, whom I did not recognize:

He raced across the room with a gasp and shook me roughly:

"My God! Ruby! What on earth *are* you doing!" he sniffed the water suspiciously, "What *are* you drinking?"

The spell was shattered, and I reverted back to the frustrated actress. With dignified head held high I stalked off to wash my face.

On my return George gave me a stern lecture: "*Never* let me see you like that again! Imagination's all very well, I know you're dippy on acting, Rubes, but you go too far. You were completely carried away . . . If you could only have seen yourself, I really thought you were dead drunk."

Shortly before this episode, my ambition and pride had received a jolt. For over a year I'd been enthralled by Henry Baynton – a Shakespearian actor, popular in the provinces at that time – and it had occurred to me that if I could watch him rehearse, my own style of acting would benefit. So I determined to talk to him next time he was in town. And so, one morning found me outside the stage door of the theatre. Two hours of patient waiting brought its reward, for there he was striding towards me; my knees turned to jelly – an agonizing wave of shyness swept over me. Nevertheless, planting myself firmly in front of him I piped out: "Good morning, Mr. Baynton."

He stared down coldly at the small figure who'd dared to confront him: "Yes?" he said haughtily.

"Mr. Baynton," I said humbly, "*please* may I come and watch you rehearse?"

He raised his hat, and replied scornfully, "I – *nev-var* rehearse." And sailed off majestically through the stage door entrance, leaving me with mouth wide open, completely crushed.

However, undaunted, the next morning once more I was at the stage door. The doorkeeper glared at me as I entreated him to allow me to have a peep into the dressing-rooms.

"It's not allowed, luv," he said gruffly. I pleaded eloquently and finally he grunted: "All right, all right . . . in and out as fast as you can, and if you're caught don't you dare say I let you in."

In a trance of rapture I wandered amongst the dusty gloominess of stage props and depressing rooms which to me seemed like paradise. Despite the previous day's snub, I almost fainted with joy when coming to the door marked 'Mr. Baynton'. Cautiously I opened the door – the room was empty. The array of greasepaints, costumes and wigs, filled me with delight. I reached out and touched one of the wigs, which unaccountably flung me into a panic . . . I rushed out of the room – straight into the arms of a tall, handsome young actor:

"Hello, hello, little girl," said he kindly, "what on earth are *you* doing here?"

"Oh, dear!" I gasped, thoroughly frightened, "er . . . I c-came in t-to see Mr. Baynton's dressing room."

"Mr. Baynton's dressing room! But don't you know no one is allowed in here? How did you get past the door-keeper?"

"Oh, well," I lied, "he wasn't there, so I just popped in."

"I see," he said, smiling at my lame excuse. "Well, now, suppose you tell me just why you were so anxious to see Mr. Baynton's dressing-room?"

"Well, you see, it's like this," I started fervently, as in the traditional style of the day I smote myself over the heart. "You see, it's the fire in here, I just *have* to be an actress, and it's vitally necessary for me to improve my style."

"Ah, so *that's* it, now I understand . . ." he lifted me up and set me down onto a barrow, then settled himself in a rickety arm-chair, and started a fatherly lecture; he drew a dour picture of the hazards of the profession; the petty jealousies, the wearying travel, dingy apartments, irate landladies, and finally; "Now, you be a good girl, go home to your dad, and forget all about acting." But I with head filled with moonbeams, rose with dignity and replied gravely:

"I just *have* to act – it's the fire you see," I held out my hand, "Goodbye, and thank you."

A year after Mother's death, George and I had a great shock, when suddenly and out of the blue Father announced his intention of marrying again. His long speech, which we listened to in dead silence, ended with: "You must know that no one can ever take your mother's place, believe me I'm doing this as much for your sakes as for my own," he turned to me, "Eirlys ought to have a mother, you know, Ruby, you've been wonderful but you're having no young life of your own – it must stop."

As we both remained dumb Father paused as he turned to leave the room and said decisively: "Nothing either of you may say or do will make me alter my mind. I'm bringing my future wife to tea tomorrow, and I want you both to make her feel welcome. She has two young sons of her own, she will be Mother to you all." Quietly and firmly he closed the door behind him.

We felt numb with shock and horror. After a few minutes pondering on the unattached ladies at our chapel, we decided that none of these had shown any such interest towards our father. George paced the room fuming: "Well," he exploded, "if he thinks I'm going to throw my arms around her neck in welcome, he's jolly well mistaken."

"It's an insult to our mother," said I, "I won't give up Lilas. I won't, I won't."

We carefully planned our conduct; George would be coldly polite, I quietly defiant. We laboured under the delusion that the lady would take our hint and depart from Father's life. Lilas went to a birthday party that afternoon and George and I waited nervously for Father's car to arrive. We fled in panic to the bathroom as it turned into the drive. When they came in Father said rather tensely to the unknown lady: "Sit in here, dear, while I call the children . . ." He called up the stairs with stern authority; "George and Ruby! Come down *immediately* for tea."

I whispered to George nervously; "You go first, George, then come back and tell me what she's like."

"All right, I'll go, but I don't mind telling you I feel awful."

I leaned over the banisters and strained my ears, but only muffled sounds of the introductions emerged from behind the closed drawing-room door. I waited impatiently for George to come up the stairs, but after a time, curiosity overcame nervousness and I gathered myself together and sailed slowly down the stairs. I expected to find George looking haughtily aloof, but not so, on opening the door a touching scene met my eyes . . . There was my brother with his arms around the lady, both were crying – so was Father.

"Treachery!" thought I inwardly fuming. I walked forward with a frigid, "How do you do?" framed on my mouth, but as I tried to speak I could only stammer, "Oh, dear me . . . " Then I too burst into tears.

Composure was restored by tea and cakes. The lady, our mother-to-be was a tall, robust handsome woman, all dimples and twinkling hazel eyes. We learned her two sons, Dick and John, respectively aged fourteen and nine, called her Dearie, and, she added it would be nice if we did the same. She was a Captain's widow from a nearby town. We learned too of the plans to transfer her furniture, cook and housemaid, over to the large house Father had bought near Hesketh Park. And later with gay farewell assurances of, "We'll meet again soon," and, "how happy we'll all be together", off they went.

George and I sank limply onto the sofa. "Really, George," said I reproachfully, "and you were supposed to be the strong, relentless one!"

He grinned impishly. "I just couldn't help myself, Rubes, she seemed so nervous, I felt darn sorry for her . . . Anyway, you were just as daft."

"Well, we've done it now," I returned mournfully, "nothing will stop them getting married."

Chapter Three

Two months later, when we were all settled in the big house, everyone tried hard to adjust to the new circumstances. It was not easy. Dearie, though a charming woman was a great contrast to the gentle mother we remembered. She, like Father, was a dominant personality and used to having her own way. All too soon their temperaments clashed. The early trouble arose over Dick, the elder son, who, maybe because of his ebullient personality, started plaguing Lilas. Tearfully, she would come running to me and show a crop of lumps and bruises, saying; "Dick did it."

The lad was a picture of innocence when tackled by his mother, and she refused to believe he did it. And then, one day he carried his pranks too far, he shut his small step-sister in a heavy chest on the landing for a lark, and quite forgot to take her out. She was discovered later – half suffocated. During the ensuing rumpus Dearie lapsed into hysterics.

None of us suspected that in spite of her tremendous vitality, she was a sick woman and subject to unaccountable attacks of acute indigestion. In my young ignorance it seemed to me that these attacks inevitably followed bouts of temper and general tension, whereas, the truth was that when they were pending, she felt so irritable she just had to fly off at someone – usually I was at hand. Father and George were away frequently travelling, and so escaped many upsets.

However, I shall always remain grateful to Dearie for persuading Father to write to Mr. Atkinson, a well-known teacher of voice in Liverpool, for an audition. Dearie had a rich contralto voice, and I a mezzo-soprano. Mr. Atkinson had a high reputation as a voice teacher, and when we received the appointment I felt horribly nervous. And thus it was, in agonies of apprehension, I found myself facing Mr. Atkinson in his studio, praying he would find my voice worth training. His grunts and murmured comments were non-committal as he made me trill up and down the scales: "Yes, yes, um – er – yes, again . . ." More trills, "Ah, sing that note again . . . again, again . . ." On and on, then two songs, after which he rose abruptly. "Thank you Miss Morris, that will do . . ."

And out he went to my Father waiting in the next room. I was thrilled when I heard him saying to Father, "Mr. Morris, your daughter has the makings of an unusually fine mezzo-soprano voice. I shall be glad to accept her as my pupil."

The thought of training with this tall, thin man with the golden voice filled me with exquisite happiness. Optimistically, I believed the door would open to the stage, and too, the weekly lessons meant adventure. And in time I found my way down to Pier Head where I would spend as long as I dared watching the great liners. Pressing my face against the iron rail I murmured over and over again: "Some day I'll sail away on one of those wonderful ships."

Time went on and the nervous tension in our home steadily mounted. I felt imprisoned, the only release from misery was my singing lesson days. Then in the second year of training I almost burst with pride when Mr. Atkinson invited me to sing at one of his concerts at the Wallasey Town Hall. Several of his pupils were on the programme including a Carl Rosa Opera star. "Tell me, Ruby," he went on, "tell me the details about that Eisteddfod, your father told me you won the first prize, I'd like to write them on my programme."

"Well," I began somewhat shyly, "I had just had my twelfth birthday and so was eligible for the eighteen-year-old's competition group. We lived in Birmingham at the time. The song was 'Bugeilio'r Gwenith Gwyn'. I can't speak Welsh, but Father drummed the words into me until my pronunciation was perfect. The Adjudicator did not know I couldn't speak Welsh until he handed me the rosette and the prize."

"How did you feel, singing in Welsh?"

"Not really nervous, but Father brags the tale of how amused the audience was at my manner on the platform . . ." I hesitated.

"Well, go on, go on, tell me all about it."

I laughed. "I suppose it was partly because I was the youngest, and so small, lost and last in the long line of girls; they all seemed so grown-up. As each girl started to sing I completely forgot the audience, I stepped forward and cocking my head towards her like a sparrow I listened intensely. Then when she finished I stepped smartly back into line smugly murmuring to myself, '*I* can sing better than that!'

"But two girls shattered my confidence. I remember thinking I couldn't possibly sing better than either of them. Apparently I looked the picture of despair, then at last I was alone on the platform."

"Were you nervous?"

"No, because I was quite lost in the mood of the song. I just sang what

I was seeing in my mind's eye, and when finished, bowed like a marionette and left the platform.

"I was shivering as I sat down by Father and listened to Welsh flowing unintelligibly around me; then when he whispered to me, 'The Adjudicator is going to name the winner of your competition now, Ruby.' I shivered even more. Soon there came cheers and loud applause, I was confused but so anxious to be a good sport I started to clap as hard as I could. Father nudged me sharply, 'It's bad manners to clap for yourself, Ruby,' he whispered excitedly, 'go onto the platform – Mr. Parry is calling *you.*' "

"I can well imagine how you looked," laughed my teacher, "Now, tell your father about the concert and next week we'll choose your group of songs, and oh, yes, I want you to ask him to drop in when he can manage it – I want to discuss your future with him. You should go to Italy for further training."

"*Italy,* Mr. Atkinson?"

"Yes, and the sooner, the better, I see a brilliant career for you, not I think for opera, I'm afraid you're too small for that, but certainly for the concert platform."

I was thrilled by the compliment, but the concert platform . . . oh, no, could no-one understand my passion for dramatic acting. I knew quite positively that there was no hope of my ever going to Italy. Our style of living was exhausting Father's resources, but even were it not so I knew nothing would induce him to let me go on the stage; his plan for me was to teach singing.

As Dearie's attacks became more frequent, anxiety deepened in our home; she was seldom free from pain. The doctor advised consultation with a Liverpool specialist. She followed the strict diet he gave her and for a time her health improved.

When George fell head over heels in love with a lovely girl who was a member of our chapel, I felt a great loneliness of heart. He was away from home a lot, so naturally he spent as many hours as possible with his beloved. I withdrew further and further into myself, determined that no-one should know the desperate misery I felt. Even though I was never involved in the strife between Father and my step-mother, I was painfully conscious of the fact that my presence in the house made life more difficult for him.

It was during this time I started my habit of humming or singing when embarrassed or upset. I went on acting the role of happy, carefree young girl. But some months later, the strain became unbearable. Constantly, my mind whirled with urgent questions: "How can I get away from home? Where can I go? What shall I do?" I had enough sense to know that running away was out of the question. I was not trained to do anything, nor had I any money of my own. But one morning, rather strangely, came the answer. I was washing my hands in the bathroom, muttering fiercely, "There's no way out, no way out at all . . . " when I suddenly heard a clear, distinct voice, stating calmly:

"You're going to hospital to learn to be a nurse."

I turned quickly, thinking someone was teasing me – no-one was there, and there was no other person upstairs at all. Slowly I went back into the bathroom and gazed into the mirror, then I addressed the pale face reflected in it: "That's right, that's what you'll do, you'll go to hospital and learn to be a nurse . . . "

And so saying, I immediately felt very sick.

When George came home, two weeks later, I told him that Father and Dearie had given me permission to go to London for an interview with the Matron of St. Mary's Hospital, Paddington. He listened to me quietly, his soft brown eyes clouded with anxiety:

"It won't work Rubes," he said tersely, "you'll never stick it. You'd be home inside three months."

"Oh, no, I won't . . . When I make up my mind to do a thing, I do it."

"I still say it won't work . . ." he grinned, "But I needn't worry – the Matron won't take a shrimp like you."

That remark flung me into earnest rehearsals of how to behave in front of a Matron of a hospital. Intuition informed me she would certainly ask: 'Why do you wish to be a nurse?' I mentally prepared a bookful of answers . . .

When the time came, due to business appointments, neither George nor Father could come with me to London; I had to face the ordeal alone. After staying a night with an Aunt in Bradford, I boarded the train at five-thirty in the morning, and settled myself in a compartment marked 'Ladies Only'. As soon as the train pulled out of the station, my acting abilities completely deserted me; I became; as indeed I was, a young girl overwhelmed by terror at going to the great city of London, and obliged to enter a fearsome hospital to be scrutinized by a Matron.

As the train sped on a sense of impending doom deepened, and bouts of 'train sickness' started. Between attacks, I rehearsed how to approach taxi-drivers, who under no circumstances should be allowed to see that I was an inexperienced 'small-town' girl. Otherwise I was quite convinced I would be whisked away to a fearful, unknown fate.

The nearer we got to London, the more frequent became my emergency exits from the carriage; the two ladies who shared it with me were eyeing me anxiously. Eventually, one of them declared firmly:

"Young lady, you look quite ill. I'm going to call the guard."

When he came, he took one look at me, then said cheerfully:

"Train sick, Miss? Soon fix that for you." He went off and soon returned with a glass of hot water and soda; "Now just you sip this, Miss," he said kindly, "you'll soon feel fine – never known it to fail."

Sure enough, by the time the train pulled into Paddington I had quite recovered. It was one of London's most depressing days; drizzle and thick yellow fog hung on the air, filling me with melancholy. An excellent setting for my mood of heroic self-sacrifice. Taxis were coming and going with what seemed to me frantic speed. Taking courage firmly in both hands I stepped briskly up to one, and addressed the driver in a loud 'do or die' manner:

"St. Mary's Hospital, Praed Street, please . . . As quickly as possible!"

The driver gave me a quick up and down look: "Right, Miss, 'op in." and we sped off into the gloom.

After paying the taxi fare, I glanced up at the formidable looking building, huge and grey; the mere sight of it made me quake. Inside the swing door I paused, wondering how I should find my way to the Matron's office. A tall, dark uniformed man with elegant waxed whiskers bore down on me, armed with all the authority of one in charge of the porter's lodge.

"Yes, Miss? Where do you want to go?"

"Would you direct me to the Matron's office, please?" I asked meekly.

He pointed towards a long corridor. "Down there and turn to the right."

My heels made a noisy tattoo along the stone floor. At the far end of the second corridor, I halted in front of an open door marked 'Assistant Matron'; I stood there uncertainly clutching Matron's letter in my hand. A few minutes later out came a lady in smart uniform: "Good morning," she said in a cool professional tone of voice.

Speechless, I held out the letter. "Oh, yes," she smiled, after a quick glance, "you are Miss Morris. Please come in and sit down. Matron will see you shortly." Presently, a bell tinkled and Sister disappeared through the communicating door into Matron's office.

Panic iced through my veins – run, flee, escape – in a minute it'll be too late – but it was too late, for Sister returned immediately and led me out into the corridor and placed me in front of Matron's door. "When the bell rings," she said quietly, "knock at the door and go in."

Praying that the earth might open and swallow me up I waited for the summons, and on hearing it, took a deep breath, knocked timidly on the door and went in. At the far end of a seemingly enormous room behind a large desk, sat a most regal figure. She wore a navy blue dress trimmed with white lace at neck and wrists, over her shoulders a navy blue cape lined with red, her crown a many frilled cap and under her chin, strings with an attractive bow. Her head was bowed over the book in which she was writing.

Like a tin soldier, stiff and erect, I approached the desk, hands tightly clasped behind my back. She went on writing. I remained silent. Suddenly, a pair of striking iris blue eyes looked up and held my gaze. Her face was pale, beautiful – the face of an angel – I promptly fell in love with her. She questioned me in a soft, firm voice, then came the inevitable, "Tell me, Miss Morris, why do you wish to be a nurse?"

A torrent of stored ideals poured forth, until out of breath I paused.

I noted a small smile creeping at the corners of her mouth; "Miss Morris," she asked with raised eyebrow, "are you quite happy in your home?"

"Oh, yes, of course I am, Matron!" I replied, in a 'how could you doubt it' tone of voice.

"I'm glad to hear it," said she gravely. She paused studying my face musingly; "Now, Miss Morris, it is important that you understand that the nursing profession is not to be undertaken lightly. Our work is hard and exacting. Before you enter the wards you will have six weeks studying in the preliminary training school, if you fail the examinations, you will of course be sent home."

"Yes, Matron," said I, in a daze.

"Your hours of duty are long – seven in the morning till nine at night. You will be entitled to two hours off duty daily, and a half-day each week. Once a month you will have a full day off, and your yearly vacation is three weeks."

"Yes, Matron."

"You will have," continued the angel, warming to her subject, "not only the hospital exams to pass, but also the Preliminary and Final State Examinations after which I trust, you will do your midwifery training. To be a successful nurse one must have a real love for nursing . . . Nursing," she added firmly, looking at me sternly, "is a vocation – do you believe it is *your* vocation?"

"Yes, Matron." I answered, almost hypnotised into believing it to be the truth.

"Very well," she rang a highly polished silver bell, "Sister will take you along to the Medical Superintendent for your physical examination."

"Thank you, Matron," trembling at the thought.

Dr. Riley was a kind young man, and I almost burst my lungs breathing "In – Out, in – out" in case he should find something wrong beneath his stethoscope. My pulse raced and I was sure he would fail me with a heart ailment. Equally certain I'd fail because stretched to the utmost – the required height of five feet evaded me. I sighed with relief as I saw him write on the report 'five feet'.

The examination over, the doctor handed the report to Sister, bade me 'good morning' pleasantly and waved us away. I resisted the temptation to bob a curtsy in thanks, instead beamed at him, "Thank you, Sir, Good morning, Sir."

Back in *the* office I watched Matron's face anxiously as she scanned through the report. She looked up and smiled. "Very satisfactory, Miss Morris. One small point though I'm afraid – I cannot take you until you are nineteen – let me see, that will be in December?"

"Yes, Matron."

She consulted a book then rang her bell. Sister appeared, "I have accepted Miss Morris, Sister, please issue her with the hospital regulations and enter her name in the book for the March School. That is our first vacancy."

She stood up, indicating the interview was over, "Now, Miss Morris, take my advice – purchase some books on practical nursing, and study. It will be much to your advantage when you enter the school." She shook hands with me; her hand was cold, frail, but seemed to possess strength of purpose. I drank in every line of her face, to store in my memory.

Outside the hospital I heaved a sigh of relief and was suddenly aware of violent hunger. Again I looked up at the huge building and looking, words from my childhood echoed in my mind, "When I grow up I'll travel and travel, but, I'll never be a nurse, I'll never marry a doctor, and I shall *never* go to China."

I hailed a taxi, thinking, Paddington station's the only safe place for me.

It seemed but a moment from the hissing departure of the train to the sound of a kindly Lancashire voice rousing me from exhausted sleep:

"Wake up, luv – wake up. We're nearly there."

By the time the train shuddered to a halt I'd fully recovered my wits. I stepped down grandly onto the platform into the arms of my family who hurled excited questions at me:

"How did you go on, Ruby?" said Father.

"Bet they didn't take you!" grinned George.

Lilas piped out as she jumped up and down, "I don't want you to go away, Ruby, I don't, I don't!"

Dearie said kindly, "You look tired, Ruby."

I replied loftily, "I'm not at *all* tired, thank you. I am *quite* all right, and of *course* she took me." Then forgetting the act, rushed on, "Oh, the Matron's an angel – I'm entered for next March, you see she can't take me till I'm nineteen, and it's the first vacancy."

"Oh, heck!" exclaimed my brother.

"Well, well," sighed Father, wiping his brow, "I don't know, Ruby, I'm afraid you'll never stick it . . . How can you? You faint at the sight of blood, and shudder when you see a doctor."

Lilas did her jumping act, "Don't go. Ruby, please, don't go."

Dearie turned on them impatiently, "For goodness sake don't be so discouraging, all of you. Of course she'll stick it – nursing's a splendid profession."

I smiled gratefully, telling myself I would not think about it, I just wouldn't . . . March was a long way off . . . Anything could happen . . . The next morning however, remembering Matron's parting words I sallied forth in Florence Nightingale mood, and took myself down to the town library. Scanning the shelves for a book on practical nursing, I finally found a tome whose illustrations so horrified me I hastily put it back and instead, chose a book entitled 'ADVENTURE IN THE AFRICAN JUNGLE'.

Early in the New Year, our step-mother fell acutely ill and was rushed back to the nursing home. A major operation was done and she was brought back by ambulance from Liverpool, still gravely ill, and needing the care of a professional nurse. The doctor sent in a heavily-starched, capable person who so terrified me I flew up and down the stairs obeying her orders, fetching and carrying from kitchen to sickroom in a constant state of 'goose-flesh'.

It was pitiful watching the once robust, handsome woman slowly fading into a wraith. The end came suddenly during another emergency operation – she died under the anaesthetic . . .

When family affairs had been straightened out, the big house brooded in heavy silence. The two boys went to live with a relative. Lilas started school and Margaret, the housemaid left to get married, leaving the cook to carry on alone.

Father and George were seldom at home. I ruminated on my future, now uncertain – uncertain until one day Father called me into his study:

a long talk about finances ended by his declaring emphatically: "Now Ruby, you must not give up the idea of nursing. It's essential that you learn a profession so you can earn a living. However," he added wistfully, "I can't let you go just yet. I'll write to the Matron explaining and ask if you can start in June . . .

And so, on the 8th of June, 1925, a shining day with the scent of lilac heavy on the air, the day of my departure from home to a new and terrifying life, I was driven to the station, the three of us upset after Lilas had gone off to school with red-rimmed eyes still protesting; "I don't want Ruby to go away, Daddy, I don't want her to go."

I leaned out of the carriage window to kiss them good-bye. Father deemed it his parental duty to repeat his awful warnings: "Remember, Ruby, my child, remember all I've told you about the white slave traffic – *Never* speak to a strange man, or woman, for that matter – under no circumstances accept a gift from a man." He hastily blew his nose, and surreptitiously wiped a stray tear from his eye.

The train pulled slowly out of the station. Both Father and Brother looked as lonely and miserable as I felt.

Chapter Four

Arriving at London I found the day still bright and shining, and after another brief glance at the address clutched in my hand, I hailed a taxi, "Twenty-three, Norfolk Square, please." The Assistant Matron's letter instructed me to present myself there at precisely three o'clock.

The taxi driver peered through his mirror, noting the white face reflected therein; "Twenty-three, Norfolk," he repeated, "that's the nurses' 'ome for St. Mary's, ain' it?"

"That's right," I responded with heart in boots.

"Well, cheer up, young miss, don't take it so hard – you'll soon get used to it. Fine 'orspital is St. Mary's – my old man died there."

Soon, we were there and my legs turned to butter as I stepped out of the taxi; while I fumbled in my purse to pay the fare, the kindly old man carried my suitcase up the five steps for me. He smiled reassuringly at me: "Thumbs up now, Miss. Don't you worry, you'll be all right."

In a fever of nervousness I rang the bell and my heart raced as I heard swift footsteps coming to the door. It opened and revealed a tall, smartly-uniformed figure which looked down at me from pale blue eyes fringed with white lashes, a mass of red hair tucked under a stiff white cap which rose to a peak like a bishop's mitre. Her lips were red and full.

Completely overcome by awe and terror I gasped out ungrammatically, "It's me – I've come!"

The eyebrows raised, "You are . . . ?"

"Ruby Morris, from Southport."

"Oh, yes, you're the new probationer. Please come in. You are the first to arrive."

I took up the heavy case and followed her into a dreary drawing-room, sparsely furnished with a round table, four armchairs and settee upholstered in black leather.

"As soon as the others arrive," said the charge-nurse, "I'll take you up to your room." She went out and closed the door behind her.

No sooner had my heart quietened down than the front doorbell shrilled, and it raced again. The charge-nurse escorted in a tall, thin girl in a black costume. Her pallor was accentuated by her black satin hat. forlornly decorated with one beige feather.

The introduction was brief. "Miss Huskinson, this is Miss Morris." Then she left us to it. We each sat on the edge of our armchair, trying to disguise shyness by gazing nonchalantly out of the window. Soon I couldn't bear the silence, so I whispered:

"Are you glad to be here?"

Her aesthetic face lit up with a charming smile as she replied raptly, "Oh, yes, indeed yes, I've waited *years* for this day. My mother is a midwife – are *you* glad?"

"Glad!" I almost groaned, "Glad? This is the worst day of my life!"

"Oh, dear," Miss Huskinson was shocked, "then why are you here?"

"Because my mother died, then my step-mother died, and now I have to be a nurse to earn my living."

"Oh, dear," she repeated lamely and lapsed into embarrassed silence.

Then Miss White and Miss Coombs joined us, Miss White of medium height and Miss Coombs every inch of six feet. With their arrival our school was complete. "Now," the charge-nurse said briskly, "come along, nurses, I will take you up to your rooms. You must be very quiet, because some of the night nurses sleep on the top floor."

Silently, we trooped after her. Miss Huskinson and I were shown into a room divided into two cubicles by a wooden partition down the centre. Neither of us spoke as we unpacked. I thought, maybe when I see that angel of a Matron I'll feel better, but I won't think about it now, I just won't.

In the early morning we struggled into our new uniform; pinstripes, starched collars and cuffs, snowy apron and bib. Long hair being the fashion of the day we were almost reduced to hysterics trying to fix the 'bishop's mitre' cap over our bun. Mine went on falling over my eyes, but eventually with much coaxing, it stayed put. Miss Huskinson marched in positively beaming with pride and joy, but I felt like a puppet dressed up for an unsuitable role. Then came the charge-nurse's strident voice from below:

"Nurses, nurses, come along! Come along at once – you're keeping me waiting!"

We flung our blue capes across our shoulders and flew down the stairs, where our two fellow nurses were already waiting. Like lost sheep returning to the fold we followed our escort over to the hospital, I walking at the side of the tall Miss Coombs. And in that order entered the nurses' dining-room in the basement; thereafter she and I were nick-named 'the long and the short of it'.

Once more my heart raced when, after breakfast the Sister Tutor gathered us together and marched us off to Matron's office. Inside, again on parade I gazed upon the face of my 'angel'. The soft, smooth voice administered a pep talk, in which she stressed the strict rule that when on duty the use of Christian names was forbidden. We learned too that as we were all young girls away from home for the first time, a late pass would not be granted during our first year. On our half-days off duty, therefore, it was imperative that we be back in the nurses' home not a minute later than ten o'clock. I rather fancied a hint of amusement in her smile as with lifted eyebrow, she looked at 'the long and the short of it'.

"Now, nurses," Matron concluded, "work hard, study diligently. After your six weeks training, I hope to have the pleasure of passing you in your examinations, and of welcoming you to the wards – Good morning, nurses."

"Thank you, Matron," we chorused, "Good morning, Matron."

The six weeks training included lectures on elementary anatomy and physiology, practical nursing, also on domestic chores that were part of our duties at Norfolk Square. In the hospital lecture room we practised practical nursing on a tortured-looking dummy named Sarah. The afternoons were occupied by writing up lectures and on alternate days, doing the domestic work and invalid cookery.

Marie Huskinson and I soon became close friends and so adopted

Christian names, but for some reason or other I started calling her Husk, or Husky, and it stuck. With our fellow students we kept to surnames.

My friend Husky soon came to the conclusion that I was *much* too young for my age, and that my head was always 'in the clouds'. She was obviously enjoying all aspects of our training; I envied the dedicated fervour in her glowing eyes and wondered miserably why I could not be like her. And then one day in the midst of a period of domestic work and alone in the study-room, my thoughts were dark with gloom, it seemed to me that all I was acquiring was a hard core of homesickness – not for Southport – but for Wales, the enchanted land of my childhood . . .

With a sigh I sank back on my heels, scrubbing brush in hand, and gazed with melancholy out through the window towards a solitary laburnum tree, a golden silhouette against the blue of the summer sky, and while gazing it faded and turned into Taid's Welsh farm . . .

And there beneath me I saw the little Chapel fach, and heard the magic music of the rill . . . I looked up to the blue haze on my favourite mountain, the Aran . . . Longing swelled up into my throat and I burst out into nostalgic singing – 'David of the White Rock'. Once started, song after sad Celtic song flowed out, then with tension easing a little I went on with the old Wessex love song. Out came the pleading words:

"Hast thou heard the turtle-dove,
When the woods are green,
Singing to his mate of love,
All his heart may mean?

So, with words as sweet as birds,
Softly I'd console.
Sing for thee, sigh for thee,
My dear soul!"

"Nurse Morris!"

The Welsh scene shattered as I was wrenched back to reality. I looked up into Sister Tutor's cold eyes:

"Very nice, very touching, Nurse Morris," said the icy voice, cold with sarcasm, "however, you are *not* allowed to sing when on duty. Now, be so good as to get on with your work."

Feeling like a deflated balloon I applied the scrubbing brush.

Although Husky was just as young and equally inexperienced as myself, she insisted in protecting me like a mother goose under a wing. Continually she reminded me that as her mother was a midwife, she was armed with knowledge of hospital routine and life in general. Wild horses would not have dragged from me the confession that my knowledge of the facts of life were hazy in the extreme. While I was aware that a baby grew within the mother, I still firmly believed the only possible exit to be through the umbilicus. No-one had told me otherwise and I never enquired. The passion for acting had left no room for curiosity on such subjects, also, in keeping with Victorian ideals, children were brought up in a woeful state of ignorance. This subject was taboo with me, I would not be drawn into it, even by Husky.

When she proudly showed me her row of medical books given to her by her mother, intimating that the mere possession of such volumes was the key to all knowledge, she then asked, "Now Ruby, let me see yours . . ." She squinted along the shelf above my bed and stared at the titles, "Shakespeare, Keats, Wordsworth, Palgraves Golden Treasurey . . . Jeffrey Farnol . . ." she turned big reproachful blue eyes on me, "Really, Ruby, and you want to be a nurse."

"I *never* wanted to be a nurse," I said hotly.

"Well, what *did* you want to be?"

"Oh, Husky! An actress, an actress!" said I, restlessly pacing the room.

"Well, then," returned my pal, prosaically, "you'd better start acting the part of a nurse . . ."

This remark set me thinking, and slowly an idea grew. I was worried about my reaction to descriptions of diseases and operations; lectures and demonstrations brought on severe attacks of nausea, and I found myself hastily retreating to the bathroom. On returning, limp and white, Sister Tutor eyed me reprovingly: "Are you all right, Nurse? You will *have* to get used to this kind of demonstration, you know."

"Thank you, Sister, yes, I'm all right – I'm sorry, Sister."

And so, during the night I worked on my inspiration. On duty, I would no longer be Ruby Morris, the romantic emotional Welsh girl; instead I would be the perfect nurse. Mentally I drew a picture of a paragon of all nursely virtues, and christened her Martha. Martha was a cool, calm, collected person, kind but firm, quite unsentimental and completely unmoved by ghastly sights and sounds. And of course she was *brilliant* at theory.

Far into the small hours I rehearsed the part, and next morning, as we walked over to the hospital, I glanced up at Husky to see if she noticed any difference in me, but all she said was:

"Oh, I'm *so* thrilled, next week we start our examinations!"

No-one at hospital ever knew of Martha's existence. Slowly, painfully, the character took shape, but 'brilliance at theory' remained a dream.

The highlight of the week's examinations proved to be my efforts at invalid cookery, which was held in the afternoon of the last day of the ordeal. The four of us stood nervously at the scrubbed table, arrayed in spotless uniform, awaiting the arrival of Sister Tutor and Matron from the hospital to supervise the effects of six weeks training. The high state of nervous tension was relieved somewhat when the 'long of it' suddenly remarked, "I wonder if Matron is psychic, and will ask Morris to make an omelette!"

This innocent remark set us rocking with laughter until tears fell down our cheeks; my efforts at making an omelette had to be seen to be believed, and the result of that examination gave me a life-long complex about omelettes.

At the sound of the front-door opening, we fought for control, and by the time the examiners came into the basement cookery room, no trace of hysterics remained, and we chanted politely:

"Good afternoon, Matron. Good afternoon, Sister."

Sister Tutor handed a paper to Matron, who came over to our table. We received our orders, mine was to make chicken broth – not too bad, I thought, surely nothing can go wrong with *that.* Back and forth we scurried, from table to back kitchen, and from table to pantry – to reach it one had to pass the ancient, unused lift-shaft and step down into the passage.

Husky's face had turned its usual shade of grey when concentrating, and my stomach was threatening the usual upheaval. Nurse Coombs on passing each other to the pantry exchanged glances, she nearly caused my undoing as she gave me a sly pat on the head and mouthed 'omelette'. After an hour of preparing the various orders, just as things were sizzling nicely on the gas-stoves, my 'angel' turned sweetly to me and said: "Nurse Morris, I would like you to make a plain omelette."

"Yes, Matron." That's done it, I thought.

I tottered into the back kitchen, blindly seeking an omelette pan. Presently, having stirred this and that together I put the mixture into the hot pan into which I had not put fat, and left it to fetch a plate. Returning, I was met by a cloud of black smoke, oh, dear, I thought and rushed to rescue my omelette, it was burnt black on the bottom and slushy on top. Fortunately, Matron was in the kitchen with her back to me; I scraped the horrid mess on the plate and hid it under my apron and headed once more for the pantry. And on passing the lift-shaft I popped the offending mess into it.

The second one turned out little better than the first. Matron gave one shocked look at it as I was putting it onto the plate, and enquired acidly: "Tell me, Nurse, if you were ill, would you care to be confronted with that?"

"No, Matron," said I truthfully.

"You are cooking for sick people, *sick people,* Nurse – make another."

Down the lift-shaft went the second omelette.

The third was nearly as bad, but at least was not burnt. Matron looked down at it, then at me, shrugged slightly and walked away without comment.

Early in the following week we were summoned to Matron's office. We formed an anxious line in front of her desk, I the midget between the tall Husky and six-foot Coombs. The Matron scrutinised our faces, then her gaze rested fondly on Husky's. She beamed at her while saying: "You have top marks in all subjects, Nurse Huskinson, I shall watch your progress with great interest. If you show the same zeal in the wards, and with your mastery of theory I feel confident you will be a credit to St. Mary's."

She left me to the last, and I quailed as one by one she turned over my papers, the mere sight of which seemed to offend her. She thumbed through them again, and I felt sick; I was convinced I was going to be sent home, a failure. Then with a slight shrug she pronounced the verdict:

"Nurse Morris, you have *just* sufficient marks for me to pass you. However, if you wish to succeed as a nurse you will have to study your theory very carefully."

The room steadied again, "Yes, Matron, thank you, Matron, I'll try hard."

And so on to the wards!

Husky's dream, and my nightmare had materialised.

Chapter Five

With fine condescension the second year nurse approached me, "I'm on Manvers – you're to come with me." With faltering steps as of one going to execution, I followed her. Up from the central hall to the top of three long flights of stone stairs where we turned left, and on to the end of the corridor. As we pushed through the swing door the ward clock struck seven; patients called out cheery 'good-mornings' as we walked down the long ward.

The junior staff nurse paused from her frantic bed-making and looked down at me, and having looked, hastily despatched me to the sluice-room; "Clean it *thoroughly,* Nurse," she ordered abruptly, "and mind it's finished by the time Sister comes on duty."

Although grateful to escape from so many eyes, the mere sight of bedpans and specimens of one kind and another made my rebellious stomach heave. When I managed to straighten up I muttered fiercely to myself, "This won't do, it simply won't do." Sternly, I ordered Martha to take over, and together we worked for an hour, to the accompaniment of despairing mutterings, "Ugh! this makes me sick, I'll never stick it . . . I'll never, never stick it."

To which Martha responded sternly, "Don't be stupid; what are you – a mouse? Don't think about it, just go on cleaning. Ignore the smells – make the place decent and shiny. There now, see how shiny and clean those bedpans look on the rack!" And I returned, "I don't care *how* shiny they look – I hate it, I hate it! Makes me sick . . . sick . . ."

Suddenly, the door swung open, "Good morning, little Nurse."

The voice startled me out of my monologue. Sister Manvers was tall and comfortably plump. Her hair was streaked with silver, and kindliness reflected from her grey eyes. She always called the new probationers 'little' until such time as they got used to her and she remembered their names.

I went hot all over, "G-good m-morning, Sister," I stammered, then brightly, "I-I've cleaned the sluice."

She ran her experienced eye round the room. "Very nice, little nurse, very nice. However," she pointed to some dark-coloured horrors on the floor, "those specimens are old – throw them away, and don't forget to wash the containers."

"Yes, er, no, Sister."

The task finished, despite Martha's scorn, I was sick again.

Every night, when Husky and I came back to our cubicles, we propped up our swollen, aching feet against a stack of pillows and exchanged the news of the day. Mostly, her conversation was a conscientious and coherent account of the medical diseases. I was quite overcome with admiration for my brilliant friend, whose every spare moment was spent with nose buried in medical books; it seemed to me she was well on the way to becoming a doctor.

My queries were a medley of requests for explanations of high-sounding medical terms and patients' idiosyncrasies. "D'you know, Husk," I started one night, "I just can't understand patients – they *are* queer. They don't complain when I splash water on the bed, nor if soap gets in their eyes, instead I'm treated to the *most* intimate confessions – usually complaints against husbands."

"Ah," said Husky with a wise look in her eyes, "you must be *firm,* you must *not* allow them to do it."

"I've tried, but it makes no difference, they go on and on . . ."

From time to time, I conveyed an astounding assortment of questions; which Nurse Huskinson stoutly declared should be put only to a priest. One woman, with tousled hair and a big floppy bosom ended her long list of complaints by asking me angrily: "Tell me, Nurse, what would *you* do with 'im? Before I come into 'orspital, I told 'im, I said, 'Now just you look 'ere, our 'arry, if yer don't leave orf doing you know what – I'll leave yer, that's wot I'll do . . .' Wouldn't *you* do the same, Nurse?"

I murmured something uncommittingly.

"An' nurse, d'yer know wot 'e 'ad the nerve to say? 'Aw, garn Nell, 'e said, 'come orf it – I've got to get some practise, haven't I?' – I'll leave 'im, that's wot I'll do . . ."

We never ceased marvelling over the questions put to us by women patients, and surprisingly by men too. We spent hours poring over books, in the hope of finding information about marital problems which we never knew existed. In time I became adept at avoiding the direct answer, by assuming an air of reserved wisdom, saying: "I'd like to think about this . . . I'll tell you tomorrow."

And quite often we'd get fed up with the search and dash out to Kensington Gardens to get away from it all.

Then when we'd been on the wards three months I made up my mind that on my day off I would sally forth to Piccadilly Circus. I had only seen Matron twice since being on the wards, and that was only the back view disappearing down a corridor. She was still an unattainable angel to me. And so, when the morning came when I had to go down to her office to request my day off I waited at the long end of the queue outside her office, in happy anticipation. As the queue shortened I noticed the rather harassed expression on the faces of Sisters and Nurses as they emerged from the inner sanctum.

I started fidgeting, then to my dismay off came a button from my sleeve . . . Oh, gosh, I thought, whatever shall I do? . . . Too late, it was my turn next . . . Oh, she'll not notice it, I'll keep my hands behind my back. I knocked at the door, entered, and as before I marched tin-soldier-like up to her desk, hands clasped behind my back. Her head was bent over a book in which she was writing, the tension in me increased with the sound of the scratching pen. Then, with a sudden jerk she raised her head and stared at me; I almost gasped out loud, for her eyes blazed with anger. Then came a razor-edged voice, she rasped out an order:

"Turn – round – Nurse Morris!"

Quivering with fright, I obeyed.

"How *dare* you come into my office with incorrect uniform?"

I tried to explain, "Well, I . . . it . . . that is, just before I came in to ask for my day off, this button came off, Matron."

"Get *out* of my office!" she roared. "When you have corrected your uniform, you may come back and make your request."

"Yes, Matron."

Outside the office I paused, thinking, it was quarter-past ten, and I knew her hour of interviews ended on the dot of ten-thirty. So I fled up to Coombs' room in the hospital nurses' dormitory, and with trembling hands, stitched back the offending button . . . I flew back to the office – just in time to see the door close. I wasted half an hour of my precious off-duty time – the door remained closed, nobody took the slightest notice of me.

Then a Welsh tantrum rose within me and I bounced off to Norfolk Square with a defiant toss of head muttering, "I won't wait longer than half an hour for *anyone* . . ." I changed into mufti and took the sorrow of my lost day off to the Peter Pan statue.

The Home Sister was waiting for me when I came out of the dining room. "Nurse Morris!"

"Yes, Sister?"

"I understand that Matron sent you away this morning to correct your uniform?"

"Yes, Sister, she did."

"Why then," demanded Sister, "Why did you not return? Matron is exceedingly angry with you!"

"But Sister," I protested hotly, "I *did* return, but the door was closed, I waited for *half an hour*," I tossed my head, "I *never* wait longer than that for any woman!"

"Nurse Morris," a little smile appeared at the corners of her mouth, "you are here for the sole purpose of training to be a nurse – the first thing you must learn is obedience. If Matron requests you to wait one hour, or twenty, then you do it. Tomorrow morning you must go to her office to apologise."

"Yes, Sister."

The rest of the day, with thoughts of the row to come, caused sudden hurried exits from the ward to the sluice room where I was horribly sick. When I finally got off duty and was walking past Matron's office to the clock room, I noticed that her door was open. On a sudden impulse I stopped and listened . . . No-one in with her . . . Why suffer like this, I reasoned, why not go in *now* and apologise, get it over with . . . maybe she'll give me my day off . . . Taking a deep breath I tapped gently on the door.

"Come in!" the voice thundered.

Once inside I took three steps forward and squeaked, "I've only come to apol . . ."

Her pale face froze with horror at the sight of a junior probationer daring to enter her office at an unorthodox hour. "*Outside* my office!" she bellowed.

Three more steps forward. "B-but, Matron – I've only come to apol . . ."

"Are you deaf, girl?" she thumped her desk, "I said *outside my office* . . . go and see my Assistant Matron!"

I hastily retreated.

I tapped at the Assistant Matron's office – no-one was there – I stood there with racing heart, wondering what to do . . . Well, I reasoned once more, Home Sister told me to apologise in the morning, so I'd better go to bed. And soon there I was warmly settled in bed, hot-water bottle on my sore stomach, and vomit-bowl handy at my side . . . Just as I was dropping off into blessèd sleep, a sudden rat-ta-ta-tat at my door jolted me awake.

The charge-nurse poked her head round the door:

"Nurse Morris, Matron wants to see you!"

I stared at her, thinking I must be dreaming, and glanced at my watch, "Now?" I gasped, "But it's half-past ten, and I'm in bed!"

"Get dressed immediately . . . Hurry, she's furious."

I threw on my clothes and feeling like a condemned prisoner, followed the nurse over to the hospital. Outside Matron's office in the cold deserted corridor, the charge-nurse whispered:

"When she rings her bell, go in." She went in to announce my presence, emerged, gave me a warm sympathetic smile and hurried away.

I waited . . . and waited . . . and waited!

When at last the bell split the silence I tottered in weakly, and in a daze of fatigue listened to the long list of my shortcomings, and the hopeless outlook of my ever qualifying as a nurse.

I'm one of those unfortunate persons seldom given to crying, but once started need sheets to cope with the deluge of tears. And to my horror I found the tears welling up and overflowing . . . And then, the miracle happened . . . Through blurred vision I saw the angry face soften into a seraphic smile! She held out both arms and cooed:

"Come here, my dear child."

In an agony of embarrassment I stumbled towards her; in my haste at dressing I'd forgotten a handkerchief, so I turned my back on her and held out my hand . . . she handed me a wispy bit of lace from her pocket to cope with the tears and sobs.

When the 'fallen angel' finally got me under control, I listened quietly to a serious talk on hospital routine, good manners, with special emphasis on hospital etiquette. Then when she'd finished, she said sweetly:

"And now, my child, go to bed – sleep well. You may have your day off."

That was an occasion when one of my angels was not popped back onto her pedestal.

Chapter Six

That encounter with Matron braced Martha into a state of wariness. She decided she was in hospital for a fixed purpose; to watch, listen and learn. Spoken words followed the monotonous pattern of, "Yes, Sister, no Sister", "Yes, Nurse, no Nurse", and "Yes, Sir, no Sir". But in between times, I hummed, trotted and patted my way round the wards.

Sunday morning routine was interrupted by a restful hour of divine service in the beautiful hospital chapel. At first, I missed the ardour of Welsh chapel-singing, in comparison, the Church of England service seemed coldly formal and correct. But gradually, I came to like the elderly dean who, in quavering tones, chanted the litanies.

When filled with women in spotless uniform, the chapel made an impressive sight. Matron, ever an imposing figure, headed the assembly, surrounded by her Sisters. Behind them came the staff nurses, senior nurses, and lastly, we probationers. To the left of the altar, the choir was made up from the seniors, and in that choir was a face which for some time had held me spellbound. A taller girl than I, with widely-spaced blue eyes, small, impudent retroussé nose, and demure mouth. Her oval, flower-like face looked idealistic. I did not know her name, but dreamed of the day when she would be my senior nurse on a ward.

Then I fell ill with tonsillitis and was sent by the Home Sister to the sick-bay, in the nurses' home. Later that evening I heard Sister saying, in the next room:

"Temperature normal again tonight, Nurse. You're much better, you may get up for a short while tomorrow."

And the following evening there came a tap at my door:

"Come in," I called huskily. The door opened – and in walked the beautiful girl from the choir! She was wearing a pretty blue dressing-gown; golden curls spread across her shoulders. I was struck dumb by joy and shyness, "Hello," she said in a most friendly way, "are you feeling better?"

I croaked: "Thank you, yes, I'm feeling better tonight."

Friendships between senior and junior nurses were sternly discouraged in hospital, but during our convalescence we shared the sick-bay sitting-room, and so it was inevitable that we should talk together, and talking led to friendship. First, there was the exchange of names: "I'm Irene Drake," she said with an enchanting smile, "but everyone calls me Rene – and you?"

"Ruby Morris, and I come from Southport."

I was enthralled when she went on to tell me that she had been born in India – someone from lands unknown!

"Father was a missionary out there for years," she went on in her soft, musical voice. "Now he's a Professor of Sanskrit at the Calcutta University. I came home to England two years ago with my two sisters."

I was still shyly reserved until the evening Rene came into the sitting-room with a book in her hand. And on seeing its title my heart leapt and every barrier collapsed:

"Oh, you too, like Keats!"

"Oh, indeed yes, and Rupert Brooke – aren't they wonderful!"

Promptly, we forgot all about seniority and indeed that we were nurses. After listening to stories about Rene's upbringing in India, I realised she was even more Victorian than myself – she was very naïve. That week of convalescence set a seal on a life-long friendship.

I went back to the wards in a much happier frame of mind. Subsequently, I discovered that being sent to a male ward was far less alarming than I'd feared. But there too, I soon found I was expected to be able to answer awkward questions. The only difference was the roundabout way the questions were put. Men with problems were apt to trail off uncomfortably into, "Well, *you* know how it is, Nurse."

One morning, after my day off, I found a new and rather different kind of patient in Bed 18. A tall young man, strikingly handsome, in an 'Ivor Novello' way. He had pleurisy, he seemed fast asleep against high-stacked pillows. As I quietly prepared to wash him, he suddenly opened gold-flecked, hazel eyes, which focused on me with a concentrated stare. Then wearily, he said:

"Good morning, Nurse." A pause, then, "Why are *you* trying to be a nurse!"

"Trying? I don't understand, Mr. –" I looked at his chart for his name.

"My name's Bill," said the patient firmly. "You look like the proverbial round peg in a square hole."

I felt rather hurt for Martha, "Oh, dear, and Sister says I'm getting on quite well – I haven't done anything wrong for some time."

"Well," returned my patient, "*don't* get soap in my eyes, and *I'll* do my hair."

Lengthy conversations with patients are strictly taboo with ward sisters, but in whispered moments during washings, and on locker and bed-castor cleaning days, Bill and I discovered that we were born within a few hours of each other, in the same month and year. And he too, from an early age had been enraptured by the words; acting, theatre, and cinema. Keats was *his* idol, and even more strange, his home circumstances had struck the death-blow to his ardent ambition to be an actor. He told me all about his friend Cliff, with whom he shared an upstairs flat in Bayswater; and I told him all about Rene.

"How very strange, Nurse Morris," he said thoughtfully, "we seem to be four of a kind."

His voice took on an even more mellow note as he described evenings spent at the flat with his sister and friends, reciting poetry, and listening to records in a room designed to shut out the hustle and bustle of London, and the harsh realities of trying to earn a living. I soon found myself seeing Cliff in my mind's eye, saw the slender, green-eyed Cliff – the nature-loving Cliff – Cliff who looked on life as a happy, endless song . . . then I lost the thread of his words and instead, listened to the rhythm of his eloquent voice:

"Come back, Nurse Morris . . ." he touched the hand poised in mid-air with wet face-cloth, "Come back, the soap's drying on my face . . ."

"Oh, dear me, I'm so sorry . . . Oh, goodness, d'you know I could almost 'see' the flat and Cliff."

"Well, look here, Nurse, you simply must meet Cliff. He'll be back from his holiday soon." He went on enthusiastically, "Why don't you and Nurse Drake come over one Sunday and have tea with us?"

I would have loved to, but I hesitated.

"Do come," urged Bill, "We'll play records and read poetry – it'll be fun . . . you will, won't you?"

Still hesitating, I said, "I'll think about it, Bill."

And in chapel, the Sunday after Bill had been sent to a convalescent home, I thought about it. In my pocket was a note with his address and scribbled directions how to reach it. I exchanged smiles with Rene in the choir, and I thought, "Yes, it's true, we four are very much alike . . ." but suddenly Father's 'warnings' swarmed and buzzed about in my mind like a hive of frightened bees . . . Two attractive young men and a flat in London added up to the red flag of danger. Although Rene was eighteen months my elder, a powerful sense of protection swept over me as I watched her sweet face.

Prudishly, I thought, 'Oh, no, I won't take her there.'

And with regret, for I thought I should never see Bill again, I tore up the note . . .

When Home Sister told Husky and me to move over to the Nurses' Home at the hospital, reminiscences of Bill, and the unknown Cliff, fell away like the falling leaves in Norfolk Square. The excitement of Christmas was filling the atmosphere in the wards. All day long scissors snipped – snapped, and shaped gaily coloured papers into patterns, bows and flowers to the designs of the Sisters and Staff Nurses. There was high rivalry on each floor between the wards; each of us trying to make our particular ward the most original and beautifully decorated.

In the midst of all the flurry, and urged on by the ever-enthusiastic Husky, I tried to concentrate on learning the circulation of the blood. It stubbornly remained a mystery to me, I could neither visualise it, nor remember the comings and goings into the ventricles of the heart.

One day when I was sitting in my room, with feet propped up, intoning, "Right ventricle . . . left ventricle . . . the blood circulates up through the – oh, dash it! Where on earth *does* it go . . . ?", there was a sudden tap on the door, and in walked Sister Tutor. I leapt to my feet with sinking heart – what *had* I done wrong now:

"Glad to find you actually studying, Nurse Morris," she said in exaggerated surprise tone of voice.

I relaxed, and waited:

"I've just come up from Matron's office – she wants to know if you will sing in the wards on Christmas Day?"

I stared at her, dumbfounded. Despite her sarcastic remarks at my outburst of nostalgic singing, she must have told Matron about the study-room incident.

"Well," she demanded, "don't stand there staring at me, girl – will you sing?"

I went hot with agitation, "Me? Sing on the wards! B-but I'm out of practice, and . . ."

"Have you any songs here?" she asked briskly.

"Yes, Sister, I have."

"Well, then, that's settled, I'll ask Nurse Pearce to play for you, she's an excellent pianist – she will arrange the times."

"Thank you, Sister," I agreed meekly.

The door closed, and I dived under my bed for my suitcase, I rummaged about until I found my tuning fork and Concone Exercise book. Hiding them under my apron I fled up to the hospital roof, and there among the chimney-tops, I tried out my voice. I was surprised to find it had not vanished through months of disuse.

Nylslie Pearce was of the same school as Rene. A tall, well-built handsome girl, with tremendous personality and Oxford accent, so overwhelmed me that I found myself singing like a mechanical doll. She was a perfect accompanist, but it was not until Rene came in as audience that the cold mood left me, the Welsh 'hwyl' flooded in and I sang for my friend. Rene too, was practising with the choir, they would do the rounds of the wards singing carols. Our off-duty times seldom coincided, so we had to be content with an occasional smile and wave of hand as we scuttled about in different directions.

The doctors and nurses did all they could to make as many patients as was possible convalescent by Christmas. They were all gay and as many as were able, helped to put up the decorations that they and ourselves had taken weeks to make. This year our ward represented a good old

English pub. At the far end stood the tall Christmas tree, decorated with red candles, bundles of sweets and a gaily-wrapped gift for each patient; and from her perch on the top branch, the mischievous-looking fairy waved her wand over the festive scene.

Before going off-duty, I pulled down the central electric lights and tied on the red 'caps'. I looked round the ward in the soft red glow, the flickering fire cast shadows, all the patients were tucked down for the night, and I felt rather like a mother leaving her children in happy anticipation of tomorrow's party.

The cheerful, "Good-night, Nurse," from the men suddenly filled me with longing for George and Lilas. It had been a long, hard day and in spite of home-sickness, I was asleep the minute my head touched the pillow.

And just as suddenly, when the harsh electric lights snapped on and the calling-up nurse sang out, "It's five-thirty, Nurse . . . Wake up, and a happy Christmas!" I was for once immediately alert. I leapt out of bed and saw snow-flakes dancing lightly against the window-pane – it would be a white Christmas.

When I'd finished my ward routine work, Sister Lewis Lloyd called me over to her desk: "Nurse Morris, Matron says that you and Nurse Pearce are going to be off duty for the rest of the day, but you must remain in uniform – you may go off now, Nurse."

"Thank you, Sister," I replied, feeling nervous and excited.

I raced up to our drawing-room, where Pearce greeted me breezily:

"Hello, Morris, sit down while I just run through my solos, then you can loosen up with your scales."

Her rendering of Liszt's 'Lieberstraum' and Macdowell's 'To a Wild Rose' was deeply sensitive, and immediately put me in the mood for singing . . . I felt the image of Martha fading out into the form of Ruby. Celtic emotion swept through me. It was Christmas Day! And we were part of the entertainment provided for the patients to try and keep their minds off the disappointment of not being at home with their families. The programme started at ten o'clock, with humorous sketches performed by the medical students. While their antics brought forth roars of laughter in one part of the hospital, the nurses' choir sang carols in the other. The big wards had a piano, and patients from the smaller wards crowded in; community singing followed after the choir left the ward.

The hospital's atmosphere of rigid discipline melted into one of easy goodwill. A blind eye was turned towards the nurses' gigglings and mild flirtations with the students. Matron and Sisters made no objection when, of necessity, I had to undo the high starched collar which choked me when I opened my mouth to sing.

There was a variety of requests for tunes and songs from the patients. For the most part the surgical cases requested cheerful songs, while in the medical wards sad songs were demanded. Almost all asked Pearce to play waltzes and medleys of Christmas carols. In Albert I sang 'All Through the Night', and as soon as I'd finished, a young man with black curly hair called out:

" 'Anwyl dad', Nurse, you have the 'hwyl'– you must be Welsh?"

As soon as I said I was he rattled off into Welsh, and looked so disappointed when I told him I could not speak Welsh, I felt like a traitor, "But I can sing in Welsh."

"Oh, Nurse, fach, sing in Welsh . . . Please sing in Welsh." So I sang 'Bwythyn Bach Melyn Fy Nhad'. Pearce rose to the occasion and managed to keep up with me. The Welshman was quite overcome and begged for more, but I had none with me.

When I'd reached the last ward I'd completely forgotten Martha, and was basking in applause from patients and warm smiles from Sister, when in walked Matron, just as I'd started another group of songs. She stood quite still while I was singing, and when I had finished, she walked over to me and, with her saint-like smile said graciously:

"You have a great gift, Nurse."

Remembering the emergency of the wispy handkerchief, I blushed to the root of my hair: "Thank you, Matron."

At the end of the long day I lay in bed while my mind floated on a sea of conflicting emotions. I was torn between fantasies of being a famous actress, and the thrill of seeing patients relax and smile, as they lay back against re-arranged pillows, or comfortable after a changed dressing: "Oh, that's *much* easier now, Nurse. Thank you, I'm sure I can sleep now."

Then at last I fell asleep as I was murmuring:

"Oh, dear me, I don't know. I suppose I'm going to spend the rest of my life being torn between Ruby and Martha."

Chapter Seven

"Ruby Morris!"

"Mmm . . . yes, Husky?" I lifted my bemused head from the book in which I was vainly trying to answer Sister Tutor's weekly test paper.

"Do you realise that we've only *three* weeks left before our hospital exams?"

"Three *weeks* . . ." I echoed, as in agitation I knocked my books off the lecture-room table, "Surely, Husk, it can't be *so* soon . . .?" I started pacing the room declaring dramatically:

"It's no use, it's no use at all; you'll have to go on alone. I haven't a hope of passing anything."

"Oh, don't be such a goose," my pal scolded, "and stop being so dramatic, you're not on the stage now. You know much more than you think and your practical marks are as good as any. But really, Ruby, how *can* you expect to get through the theory unless you study your lectures *every* day . . . Don't you want to pass?"

"Oh, yes, I do, I do, but it – dash it all, Husk – I just *can't* keep awake. The minute I start reading the circulation and the liver, I fall asleep – I'm so *tired*." To prove it I yawned widely and heaved a sigh.

"Really, Ruby, you make me cross," though she laughed as she stooped to pick up my books, wrinkling her nose in horror as she looked at my awful handwriting, "Just *look* at all these blots, and your spelling . . . !"

She read on down the page and suddenly gave a snort of disgust:

"Just listen to this! 'The patient should be treated for shock by covering him with warm blankets, and placing near him covered hot-water bottles. The doctor would admit *him* to the gynaecological ward for immediate surgery . . .' Oh, quite honestly, Ruby, don't you *know* the gynae ward is for *women's* diseases?"

"Oh, Great Scott!" said I, quite shocked, "*so* it is. Now I *did* know that, Husk . . . it just goes to show how tired I am!"

"Now look, Ruby dear," said Husk patiently, "you'll just have to forget about being tired. What about Rene – she's a gold medallist, don't forget, you can't let *her* down, can you?"

This remark struck the target for I had said nothing to Rene about my boredom at reading theory.

"I tell you what," my friend went on after a moment's ruminating, "I know what we'll do . . . we'll ask Rene to loan you her first year lecture books. You study them and I'll question you every day."

"Mmm, a good idea I suppose, but you know half my trouble is, Husk, that I'm only really interested in psychology and mesmerism."

She gave a huge grin, "That's all very well, and I know all about your gift for handling loonys, but *that's* not going to get you through all the exams. Think of it – three weeks!"

The very thought made me shiver; it was all very well for my dedicated friend, who was immediately in some seventh heaven the minute her nose was dipped into a medical book. I was quite sure that she too would be a gold medallist. I thought, ruefully, it would just be my luck to have two such brilliant friends to try to keep pace with. Our school was now reduced to just the two of us, as Nurse White suddenly left the hospital, and the 'long of it' decided she preferred Charing Cross Hospital. And so, Sister Tutor had told us we would be sitting for our exams with the school that followed ours.

Rene's lecture books were models of perfection; clear, strong handwriting, free from blots – I read them until my head swam. Both my friends were determined to push me through the first-year exams, and at every opportunity dinned into my ears a medley of answers to questions that might appear in the exam papers.

The dreaded week was faced in a state of acute nervousness, which frequently erupted into awful attacks of stomach cramps. This affliction became a joke with my fellow nurses, and the answer to the query, "Where's Morris disappeared to?", was, "Oh, off to the usual – just seen her disappearing with hands over tum . . ."

As I expected Husky emerged triumphant – top marks in all papers and was congratulated by Matron herself. I achieved a bare pass in all save the medical paper, which I failed miserably. I was summoned to Sister Tutor's office. With the butterflies fluttering about in the usual way, I knocked feebly at her door. Inside, she treated me to an icy stare . . . How *could* it be that one of *her* students should get such low marks:

"Good morning, Nurse, I trust you feel quite satisfied with the results of your exams?"

I turned crimson and remained dumb.

She brought out the medical paper: "This is an absolute disgrace. Will you *ever* learn the circulation? I'm quite ashamed of you – it's sheer laziness, you know. You are a very good practical nurse, but you have to use your brain, Nurse, your *brain.*"

"Yes, Sister."

"You cannot qualify until you've passed every exam, and that means hard and conscientious study. Remember, you are here for one purpose – to qualify as a nurse. And unless you stop dreaming, I can see no hope of you ever receiving your certificates."

"I'm sorry, Sister, I'll try, Sister."

Unexpectedly, she relented and smiled kindly at me, which made me feel even worse:

"All right, Nurse, run along . . ."

I blinked back hot tears and turned to go, but she said: "Cheer up, Nurse Morris, I *know* you can succeed. If you try you can become a first class nurse . . . Don't let me down, I like to feel proud of my students."

By now, my friend Huskinson and I flattered ourselves that we were experienced 'city girls'. This meant of course that we were able to find our way on the underground to Piccadilly Circus, and back again, without getting lost. This adventure we shared on our days off, that is, when we could afford it. Pay-days came at three monthly intervals, and as our salary was fifteen pounds in the first year, rising to the princely sum of eighteen pounds in the third year, it was not so often we could afford the exciting outing.

Always, our rendezvous was the second floor of Lyon's Corner House, Piccadilly. Nor did our off-duty days coincide often. My routine was to go to a table for two, then place my coat and handbag on the other chair in the hope of discouraging anyone from joining me, and thus break in on my reveries. There I'd sit, very prim and straight in the chair and give the 'nippy' the order that never varied . . . a plate of brown bread and butter, please, with strawberry-jam, china tea and a slice of Dundee cake . . .

This I made last out for about two hours while listening to the orchestra. The conductor was a tall man with a mane of fine, blond hair. And with wild flourish of arms, he extracted every ounce of syrupy emotion from the men under his baton. The swaying, sighing and weeping of the violins fired my imagination – Martha vanished, and Ruby indulged in story-making. I saw visions of pathos, humour and tragedy in the faces around me. The stories became so real to me that, on sometimes seeing the same faces again, I would add another chapter according to their expression.

The highlight of those days of escape was going to the New Gallery Kinema in Regent Street, where the surfeit of emotion was augmented with the adventures, joys and sorrows of those days – Ronald Colman, Vilma Banky and Gary Cooper. Only on one occasion my father's 'warnings' came to pass – walking down Regent Street, en route to the Corner House, I suddenly was aware that a man was following me. My heart threatened to stop beating as with a sweep of imagination I saw white slavers scooping me up, and whisking me off by taxi to some horrible unimaginable fate:

How to shake him off?

I tried gazing into shop windows, hoping to tire him out, but when I moved, so did he. I thought, now if he speaks to me, I won't say a word, not one word . . . One word leads to another – I'll just *look* at him!

Then, sure enough, right by the cinema, he drew level with me and said enticingly, "Good afternoon, Miss – care for a walk?" I turned to him sharply and stared into his eyes and walked on in silence. He repeated his invitation, and I went on staring into his horrible red-brown eyes. Eventually, he actually flushed, and mumbled, "Must be dumb. All right, all right – don't get your hair off." He raised his hat, turned away and disappeared.

It was always a struggle to call up Martha after a day off. And at the end of our first year, when the lilacs bloomed again, each day was an eternity of waiting, waiting for the longed-for moment when I would board the train that would take me on three weeks wonderful holiday – to Wales. Once more family circumstances had changed. Father had married again; this time the event caused no emotional upheaval for neither George nor myself. For our new stepmother was a member of our family – a second cousin and my namesake, my second name being Margaretta. Margaretta Morris, a headmistress to a girls' school in South Wales, had always been my favourite relative. She resigned her post to marry Father, and they were now settled in Prestatyn, including Lily, the cook, who had gone along with them.

As the time drew nearer my need to get away from hospital with its burden of human suffering, became almost a frenzy. Even the light humorous moments, and of these there were many in the wards, did not help me much. I was always conscious of the anxiety behind the cheerful patter of patients' visitors.

The Welsh hills were a beckoning paradise of escape; there I could roam alone for three whole weeks, and try to forget the ill-fitting pattern into which I had determined to train myself. And yet when the moment came and I tumbled almost at the last minute into the train, bits of my heart were left behind with Rene and Husky who came to see me off. The guard blew his whistle; the train started to move, Rene called out:

"Write to me, Ruby, and mind you come back!"

"Mind you *study* . . ." the ever practical Husk called out, "or you'll forget everything in three weeks . . ."

Three weeks in Wales!

Down through the years, going back to Wales means going home! There's a welcome in silver lake and gurgling brook, in every hill and valley, there's a welcome in the warmth of Welsh voices. And always, when the train crosses the border my cheeks flame with excitement, and I have to hold on to myself not to cry out:

"It's me! Here I am again . . . I'm home!"

When the train drew in at Prestatyn station, the first person I saw was an excited 'leggy' little girl staring up intently at the carriages – my sister Lilas! As soon as she caught sight of me she raced along the platform shouting:

"Daddy, Daddy, there she is! There she is! Ruby's come home – oh, goody, goody, goody . . ."

And as I stepped down onto the platform she flung herself into my arms, chirping merrily. Father and my new stepmother came up at a more respectable pace and greeted me affectionately. Father searched my face, "Are you happy at hospital, Ruby? Somehow your letters don't quite convince . . ."

And I, being almost delirious with joy lied convincingly:

"Oh, of course I like it, Dad, but it's wonderful to come home to Wales."

I fell in love with our new home set below Prestatyn hill, the garden was a riot of colour, for Father, besides being a water-diviner, had green fingers – every plant he touched, flourished.

Although welcoming Father's marriage I felt a little shy at first, not knowing quite what to call her. I had always called her Gret, as the family and her friends did. Now Lilas was calling her 'Mother'. It was not until she came up to my room and started rather shyly, "Ruby dear, I hope my marrying your father was not a shock to you . . ." she turned away and made a gesture of straightening a curtain, then went on quietly, "I don't expect you to call me 'Mother' – I would rather be your friend."

I ran to her and hugged her. "Oh, Gret, you *know* you've always been my favourite person, you've always seemed my friend, I'm *glad* you married Dad. You know I love you."

In those days, and even now, I'm in awe of people with academic accomplishments. I was bitterly disappointed at not being able to go to college and university. Gret had been one of my God-like people and in her presence I was usually speechless. But now all that had gone, and I felt at ease with her. And so, one day I confided to her the vagaries of my squeamish stomach. It was such a relief to talk to someone about it:

"Everything seems to make me sick, Gret. The sight of wounds makes my flesh creep, smells nauseate me, and I can't bear seeing the sufferings of people, especially the children . . . What have *they* ever done to deserve suffering . . .?"

"You'll get used to it, Fach," said Gret soothingly.

"I hope you're right, Gret, but unfortunately, that's not the whole trouble. I just cannot see myself passing all those exams. I find studying hard, worse still, it bores me stiff."

Gret started pounding common sense into my head. "All studying is hard, Ruby. I *hated* it, and I had to work much harder than the others. We all had to earn our own living. Tada drummed that into us all when we started school – what else could he do with nineteen children?"

"Yes, but Gret," I protested, "*you* went on with your schooling. I went to nine useless private schools and left before I was fourteen – oh, I feel so ignorant!"

"Well, I can tell you one thing, Ruby, I've taught girls all my life and I know ability when I see it. I assure you, Ruby, if you make up your mind, you *can* do it."

"Maybe you're right, Gret, I hope so, but in any case there's no escape – I've got to go on."

But it was to George that I looked forward to unburdening the full tale of woes. He alone, knew what giving up the ambition for the stage had meant to me. And so when he arrived, a day earlier than expected, I flew down the stairs and flung myself into his comforting arms:

"Hello, hello, love, and how are you?" he said in his Lancashire accent, "Let's look at our nurse from London . . . hmm . . . not too bad," he held me at arms' length, his warm brown eyes twinkling as he scrutinised my face, "Well, they've not killed you yet then?"

I opened my mouth to speak but Lilas rushed downstairs; she sprang into his arms, singing her usual little theme: "George has come home. George is here! Oh, goody, goody goody . . ." When he put her down she bounced up and down like a brown ball, chanting, "When I grow up I'm going to be a nurse, just like Ruby."

"Oh, you are, are you, love? Well, you'll have to grow tall, they like tall, strong girls in hospital – not a shrimp like your sister, Ruby."

"I'm *not* going to be tall," said the small girl stoutly, "I'm going to be just like Ruby."

George too was very attached to Gret, and we all felt at ease in our new home. He always radiated fun and gaiety, it was hard to be near him without feeling it was good to be alive.

The day before my brother came I had roamed the hills, up and down dale, delighted at the sight of fleeting rabbits, bobtails a streak of white as they dived into the safety of their burrows. In Wales, neither wind, mist, nor rain ever quelled my spirit. Up above the mountain-top and far into the sky it soared. Birdsong, rustling leaves and fragrance of flowers set my throat athrob, until the sheer joy of life made me burst into song:

> "I love life, I love life;
> I want to live, drink of life's fullness –
> Take all it can give,
> *I love life*."

But this time, after a while my morale began to flag. I tried to banish depressing thoughts; I murmured aloud "time enough to think about it all when I'm on the train".

On the last day of my holiday, George and I went to Dyserth and strolled around the haunts of our childhood, for nearby Rhyl had been one of our nomadic changes. During enchanted summers we three children were forever wandering about with picnic baskets in hand, George seeking a river in which to fish; as he was my alter ego, I trailed behind him proudly bearing his precious tin of bait. While Rossie, our faithful guardian laughed and frisked about in Doggy ecstasy, her mouth watering at the heavenly scent of rabbits which she always failed to catch.

While George stood in monumental patience waiting for a lethargic fish to rise for his bait, Rossie would sit meekly while Cassie and I draped round her, garlands of buttercups and daisies; she was quite used to being dressed up as a baby and taken for 'walks' in my doll's pram.

We came to a well known spot and sat down, almost expecting Rossie to come running eagerly to us. Here it was that one fearful day she had taken a fancy to George's bait. He'd put a succulent piece of fish on the wicked-looking hooks, and while his back was turned, Rossie crept up and swallowed the lot, and when George lifted the rod, there to his horror was Rossie firmly attached to the other end.

He cried out frantically:

"Cassie, Ruby – come quickly! Oh, what *shall* we do – Rossie has swallowed the hooks!"

We rushed to him, and Rossie looked up at us in mute appeal. Her bobtail drooped sadly, her big eyes were full of guilty fear. I started sobbing; "Oh, she'll die, she'll die . . ."

But George immediately took control of the situation:

"Shut up, Ruby," he ordered, "you'll make her panic . . ." He stooped down and smoothed her head and spoke quietly to her, "Good girl,

Rossie, good girl – sit down, open mouth."

She obeyed, and to our horror there was no sign of the hooks, her tongue was cut and bleeding. George cut the line and we ran all the way home . . . After the administrations of the vet Rossie was none the worse for her adventure.

And now, as we watched the river flowing serenely at our feet, we became melancholy. George gave a sudden, abrupt sigh and jumped to his feet: "Come on, Rubes, let's go . . . No use brooding, one can't put back the clock." We walked on, hand in hand, talking about his plans for his coming marriage with Muriel, his one and only sweetheart. It was a bitter disappointment I could not be there for it. "Cheer up, Rubes, you'll be seeing us in London – we're coming up for our honeymoon."

I cheered up, "Oh, gosh, George, how lovely, that means too you'll both be able to meet Rene and Husky."

George stopped in his tracks and eyed me searchingly:

"Now, come on, tell me – just how is it with you at the hospital?"

"Oh, so so . . ." and tried to change the conversation.

"Now then, my girl, you know you can't fool your brother George . . . You're finding it grim, aren't you?"

So out it all came . . . the nausea, the tiredness, the boredom: "Sometimes, George, I think I just cannot stick another minute of it."

He gave me a knowing look:

"Does that mean you're still goofy about the stage?"

"As bad as ever," I admitted, "but I do try not to think of it."

We walked on for a time in silence. Then George turned to me with understanding eyes, as he said: "You know, the trouble with you, Rubes, is that you're forever chasing the rainbow and crying for the moon."

"You mean my 'topsy-turvy' moods?"

"I mean your over-active imagination," he grinned. "You want drama, with a capital 'D'. Well, love, dash it all, if that's what you want, surely there's enough drama in a hospital to last you a lifetime?"

"True enough, George, it's dramatic all right, but the trouble is Sister Tutor keeps on telling me I have to use my brain! And when it comes to studying, I'm afraid I haven't any . . ."

"Don't be so daft, Ruby, you've got a complex over that because you had to leave school so early. Mother's death messed things up for all of us. You've jolly well got to take this as a challenge . . . You've always hankered after degrees, haven't you? Well, now's your chance to get some qualifications."

But in the glory of that summer day it was hard to believe I'd soon have to link up again with my shadow, Martha.

"O.K. George, I'll stick it and I *will* pass those exams . . . somehow or other . . ."

And there and then I resolved, come what may, I would *get* those certificates.

All the family came to see me off at the station next day.

Dad and Gret smiled encouragement, Lilas waved forlornly, and as the train pulled out, George grinned and called out:

"Good old Rubes . . . Remember our motto – Up the Morris's!"

"That's it," I laughed, "That's it . . . Up the Morris's!"

Chapter Eight

"So you *did* come back, after all," Husky greeted me cheerily, "I really had my doubts, you know," her puckish grin deepened, "no need to ask if you're glad to be back – you look as though you're facing a life sentence . . . Have a good time?" She was busy unpacking.

"Every minute was wonderful – Wales always casts a spell over me . . ." I pulled myself together sharply, "Sorry, Husky love, I'm not quite back – did you have a good time?"

"S'spose so," she admitted vaguely, "I felt horribly tired at first, so I just sat around; studied a lot and gave Mum no peace when she came in from her 'midder' cases. I now know *all* the positions of the baby in relation to the mother – bet you didn't open a book!"

"Heavens, no, Husk, I didn't even take one with me. I *know* I shall simply detest midwifery, but thank goodness I don't even have to think about it for two years."

"Never too early to learn, my girl," my brilliant friend assured me loftily, "Anyway, I shall love it." She scrutinized me keenly, "Now come on, Nurse Morris, snap out of it, down from those clouds, and unpack. Rene will be back next week, and you can drool over your beloved Wales with her." No risk of my feet not being encouraged to keep firmly on earth when Husky was about.

I longed to see Rene, for although she was a born nurse, she was also an incurable romantic, and would listen to my raptures.

Next morning, bleary-eyed and half awake we trotted down to breakfast, wondering what our fate would be. Nauseated by the mere sight of the huge platters of fried eggs and greasy-looking bacon, I mumbled: "Good morning, Sister. I don't want anything to eat, thank you."

"Oh, yes, you do, Nurse Morris, you know quite well by now that you are not allowed on the wards without taking breakfast," she looked hard at me, "Are you sick?"

"No, Sister, I'm not sick."

So I was handed a loaded plate; I wended my way through the maze of tables to sit beside Husky who was tucking in heartily. After breakfast came Sister's announcements – we received a shock when our names were read out to move over again to Norfolk Square. This meant we were going on night-duty – Husky on Lewis Lloyd, I on Manvers. We hurried back to our room to pack, and I felt a strange sense of relief at going on night duty, it seemed an escape from the grim realities of the day. We carried our suitcases over to the Square and heaved them up to the top floor. Again we were lucky, we were sharing a room. As we unpacked, cheery giggles and squeals came from the other bedrooms, where the night-nurses were changing into mufti.

We had to be in bed by twelve o'clock; it was a lovely day so we went to our usual seat by Peter Pan statue and fell to ruminating; said Husky, "Imagine, Ruby, we shall be night-birds for three whole months. Just fancy having to sleep away all these glorious days!"

"Oh, I don't mind," I returned gloomily, "If I can't be at home, I may just as well sleep all day and work all night . . . but what luck getting Manvers."

"That's only half of it – you're getting Nurse Gallagher as senior, she's wonderful. I don't know Lewis."

"Oh, bother," a sudden thought struck me, "we won't be able to go to the Corner House until we get our nights off."

"I'm lucky too, living in Denham I can get home for mine."

"Lucky you," a wave of home-sickness enveloped me, "Oh, dash it, let's go and have coffee."

The first week on night duty passed in a perpetual daze of fatigue, then as we got used to the routine we began to enjoy it. Husky liked Lewis, and Nurse Gallagher filled me with awe, and inspired me to try to emulate her saint-like qualities. A tall, slender girl with brown hair and grey eyes, the daughter of a Quaker family. No matter what the circumstances I never once saw her flustered, nor in a hurry. She worked in a slow, methodical way, was firm but ever gentle with the patients *and* her junior nurse . . . she was all I had dreamed Martha would become – a perfect nurse.

Steadily, I grew more and more like a broody hen – on duty and off. I worried about the patients. They intruded on my day-time sleep in nightmare fashion. I saw them swallowing the wrong medicine, falling out of bed, or screaming with pain, especially the children. And at times when I wakened shouting, "Husky, stop him! Husky, save her . . . Husky, she's falling . . ." my patient friend would leap out from her bed to quieten me with soothing words . . . "It's all right, dear, it's all right, you've been dreaming again . . . Quiet now, go to sleep . . . you're all right."

And then, gradually, I developed an impression that 'something' hovered about the ward during the night. At first I thought it might be caused by the eerie glow from the 'red' caps that were used in those days to cover the lowered lights, or perhaps from the stillness of the sleeping patients. But my uncertainty disappeared when one night, a patient to whom I was very attached, died . . . Mrs. Downer had been desperately ill with abdominal cancer. The operation had done nothing to relieve the condition. She was dying. Once a beautiful woman she was reduced to a mere skeleton, from which bulged a monstrous belly. Her gaunt, tortured face retained an expression of indescribable sweetness, and infinite patience reflected from her luminous, green eyes.

I was full of rebellion over her prolonged suffering . . . In the night I stormed within myself, "Why should such a lovely person – or, for that matter, anyone – be allowed to suffer so abominably and die so slowly?" To me it seemed we were officiously keeping her alive. On several occasions it seemed the end had come . . . But each time, everyone rushed to their duties – heart stimulants, brandy and oxygen would be administered to coax life back into the reluctant body – red screens round the bed – the house surgeon hastily summoned. This went on for two long weeks.

Then one night when we came on duty, it was obvious nothing would restore Mrs. Downer, she would die before dawn. Mercifully unconscious she lay back against her stack of pillows. At two o'clock her breathing changed to Cheyne-Stokes, the awful sound of approaching death. While Nurse Gallagher went to phone for Night Sister, I stayed at the patient's side. She started moaning and rolling her head. Hoping she could hear me I held the wasted hand, and whispered, "Don't be afraid, dear, don't be afraid . . . Sister is sending for your children."

Suddenly, she gave a sharp gasp, her eyes opened wide – she was fully conscious and alert. Without warning she sat bolt upright from her pillows and stared steadily over my shoulder – a shiver shook me, and I involuntarily looked over my shoulder – no-one was there. The patient went on staring, staring . . . Slowly, the haggard features registered an expression of absolute incredulity; then her face softened into a smile of intense joy . . . in all my life I've never seen a more beautiful smile. Then she said in a loud, clear voice:

"Oh! *I – never* – thought – that – *you* – would . . ."

She gave a gasp and fell back against her pillows – dead.

It was during those first three months on night duty that I found myself becoming very sensitive to the auras around patients, and people in general. Often, when hopes were high for a patient's recovery, I *knew* that he, or she, would die; this intuition was seldom wrong, and I spent many hours during the long night pondering about this growing awareness. One night when Gallagher and I were sitting in the kitchen having our midnight meal, I saw my senior nurse watching me closely with her calm eyes:

"What's the matter, Morris! You seem to be in a brown study!"

"Do you ever get queer feelings about patients, Nurse?"

"Queer feelings . . ." she repeated seriously, "What kind of queer feelings?"

"Umm . . . I don't know really how to express it . . . queer, shivery feelings. Many times I know almost exactly when a patient will die, and I sense 'people' round the bed."

She laughed kindly, "Oh, go on with you, Morris, you're such a dramatic little thing . . . You let your imagination run away with you."

"No, Nurse," I protested solemnly, "it's not imagination – I don't understand it at all, and what's more I can tell you I don't like it."

She laughed softly again, "You remind me of Nurse Jones – *she's* always swearing that she sees a blue light round a baby's head just as it's born. Must be the celt in you!" She got up abruptly, "Anyway, Nurse, the best cure for such thoughts is to work and study hard." She turned away and went back into the ward.

On one hectic night we had two emergencies in quick succession. The second was a fat woman with red hair; she was in great pain and as we prepared her for the theatre she groaned horribly. The operation was successful, but she was too ill for several days to take any interest in the doings of the ward. She was an Englishwoman with a foreign name, Mrs. Aben Nezra. Apart from her name there was something unusual about her. She maintained she was psychic; she became very popular with the day nurses because, in Sister's absence she read hands and when possible, the cards also.

When we came on duty at night, the day nurse passed on small items of gossip – it appeared that Mrs. Aben Nezra's husband was living in Cairo, and her one and only visitor was a coal-black gentleman who glided mysteriously into the ward, spoke politely to her for a few moments, then glided away again.

For some reason she took a fancy to me, and the day before her discharge from the hospital, gave me a hearty invitation to come to her home for lunch. The address she handed to me was a fifteen minute bus ride from the hospital; the house too, had a foreign name. Sensing my hesitation she urged me: "*Do* come, and bring along a friend . . . I'll read the cards for you both." I said I'd try to come two weeks hence, on Sunday, when I was due for two nights off.

When I told Husky about it she snorted indignantly. "Don't you *dare* do any such thing, Ruby, from what you've told me about that lady there's something queer about her."

But Rene, ever ready for adventure was enthusiastic:

"I'll come with you, Ruby, it sounds most intriguing, I'll come like a shot if I can get the day off."

"Oh, well," I said in deference to Husky's fear, "perhaps I won't go . . ." But I knew I would.

And on the day, Rene could not get the day off, so I went off on my own, in spite of her begging me not to; "Don't worry, love," I said with more confidence than I felt, "It'll be quite all right," but I giggled a bit nervously, "If I'm not back by supper-time, you'd better tell Matron where I went."

At about eleven-thirty I sallied forth and hopped onto a bus. Arriving at the street, I wandered about until I came to the house – a gloomy place. I strolled past it several times before plucking up enough courage to ring the bell. When I did so it tinkled hollowly at the back of the house. In a few moments the door opened a few inches, revealing a slovenly-looking maid. There was a hint of brogue in her voice: "And what would you be after?" she demanded.

"I'm Nurse Morris . . . Mrs. Nezra is expecting me."

"Oh," said the girl in a non-committal voice, and shuffled back to the foot of the stairs and shouted out shrilly: "Mrs. Nezra, mum!"

"Yes, Rosalie, what is it?" came a distant voice, presumably from the bathroom.

"There's a girl at the door – says she's Nurse Morris – would you be after expecting her?"

"That's right, Rosalie, show her up to the drawing-room. Tell her I'm having a bath, will you? I won't be long."

Rosalie came back and opened the door wide: "She says it's all right, you're to come up."

Inside, a smell of stale cabbage-water hovered sickeningly in the air. I followed the down-at-heel Rosalie, heartily wishing I had not come. A sharp right turn and up three more steps brought us to the drawing-room. Rosalie opened the door, I walked in and she slammed it shut behind me.

A hot wave of panic swept over me, for standing by the fireplace were two men, both foreigners. The shorter of the two, a good six feet, was a negro; the other looked Egyptian and wore a goatee beard. They were conversing in some foreign language. I was so terrified I thought my heart would stop beating, and I trembled from head to foot . . . *Now* you've done it, I thought, you've certainly done it . . . My legs just wouldn't support me and I sank on the couch opposite the door . . . I had another hasty look at them . . . No doubt about it – WHITE SLAVERS.

But the two men took not the slightest notice of me, and went on with their animated conversation. My hopes rose – perhaps one of them was the elusive Mr. Nezra. Trying to appear a woman of the world, I rummaged in my bag and took out a letter from George. But I couldn't stop the pages trembling. Soon a few rapid sentences sounded like farewells . . . Then the two men bowed politely to each other, and the bearded one without so much as a glance at me, walked gracefully past me, out of the room, closing the door behind him.

I was alone with the negro!

My eyes misted over with terror as he came towards me slowly, and when he looked down at me I could scarcely see his face . . . Oh, dear, I thought, I'm going to faint.

He bowed and said in stiff, over-correct English:

"I think perhaps, you are waiting for Mrs. Aben Nezra?"

"Yes," I replied in a tiny voice.

"She will not keep you waiting long – I think."

He bowed again and left the room.

Then in came Mrs. Nezra, bustling and gushing apologies for being in the bath when I arrived; "Still weak, Nurse dear," she puffed, "can't seem to pick up somehow." Her red hair was a mass of tight curls.

I took a quiet breath of relief and waited for the explanation of the two men – none came, instead she said, "Don't sit there, Nurse, come to the fireplace, much more cosy here." We sat facing each other and she chatted away cheerfully about her emergency to the hospital. No mention was made of the missing Mr. Nezra. All the time I waited, after each pause, for her to tell me what those men were doing in her drawing-room. But she seemed unaware that they had been there. Just as I was wondering if I'd had an hallucination, the door opened and in walked a woman with short, frizzy hair – a negress.

Mrs. Nezra greeted her with a broad smile, then made brief introductions, "This is Nurse Morris from St. Mary's Hospital," she said. I did not catch the woman's name, which sounded unpronounceable. So I smiled a polite "How do you do?"

"Nicely, thanks," she returned with a shy smile.

During the next half-hour several men and women wandered in and out, all were coloured. Mrs. Nezra kept up animated conversation, though no mention was made about card-reading. Eventually Rosalie poked her head round the door, announcing briefly:

"It's on the table, mum."

"Coming, Rosalie," our hostess heaved herself from her chair, "Come along, dear, you must be hungry – nurses always are."

We trooped after her down the stairs, and went into a spacious, high-ceilinged dining-room, in the centre of which was a long table.

Mrs. Nezra seated herself at the head of the table and motioned me to the other end. In a few minutes every place was filled. I felt rather like 'Alice in Wonderland'. Until then my only contact with people of other races had been through books.

I was completely enthralled. To my fevered imagination it all seemed wonderfully mysterious. Lunch continued more or less in silence, as they all seemed shy. When remarks did come forth, the halting English and accent made it difficult to understand them. I thought them naively charming. But nothing was said that gave me a clue as to who or what they were. At last one by one they rose, came over to me, gravely shook hands and departed.

I looked at Mrs. Nezra thinking, surely now she will tell me something about them, but no, she went on chatting lightly about nothing in particular. When I deemed it polite to leave, I got up and thanked her for the lunch:

"I've *so* enjoyed having you, Nurse dear," she crooned, "You *will* come again, won't you? Got so *much* to tell you . . . My husband you know, he . . ." the sentence trailed away with a vague gesture of her hand.

So I bade her 'goodbye' inwardly deciding never to come here again. I suffered a surfeit from confidences about 'husbands' at hospital. To be exposed to such tales of woe on my off-duty hours was more than I could bear. But I was delighted with the foreigners, and my determination to travel the world and meet its peoples was strengthened.

Although we'd enjoyed the novelty of night duty, we were both glad when it ended. Husky and I were lucky, unlike some of our fellow nurses who found it hard to sleep during the day; we usually slept soundly. Indeed, sleep was responsible for an uncanny incident that happened on our last night on duty . . .

In the room next to ours, two nurses who were close friends, Nurse Smith and Nurse Storey, overslept. They were both very reserved and excellent nurses. On this particular night, Husky and I were rather late jumping out of bed. And having flung ourselves into uniform, just as we left the bedroom we heard Storey's voice:

"Wake up, Nora, wake up," she was saying urgently, "Whatever is the matter with you? Wake up, *wake up*."

We dashed over to the hospital, and got into our places at the breakfast table, just before Sister came in. Ten minutes later, Storey came in, out of breath and upset:

"I'm so sorry I'm late, Sister," she gasped, "but I just could not waken Nurse Smith. She's awfully upset, Sister, she'd had an awful dream, Sister, it was so vivid she's terrified. She'll be over soon. Please don't be angry with her, Sister, she's so upset."

"Very well," she replied, kindly, "you may sit down."

Nurse Storey's place was opposite ours in the centre of the table. She told us the details of the dream.

A dream within a dream; Smith dreamt she could not wake up. Someone was shaking her, insisting she would be late for breakfast. In the dream she struggled to wake up, and managed it but was late for breakfast. She apologised to Sister, sat down at table, and took up her knife and fork. Just then the door opened and in came a maid, a telegram in her hand. This she handed to Sister, who quickly opened it, and as she read it, a look of concern crossed her face. She looked up at Smith: "It's about you, Nurse, I'm afraid it's bad news from home . . . Matron knows about it and I'm sure she will arrange for you to get home as soon as possible . . ." She passed the telegram over, "Go now to Matron . . ."

Storey broke off as Nurse Smith came into the dining-room, looking deathly pale. She apologised to Sister, took up her knife and fork . . . A loud knock at the dining-room door made us all start and sit up stiffly. In deathly hush, every head turned to the door.

Exactly as in the dream, in walked a maid, a telegram in her hand. She took it straight to Sister who opened it, read it, then looked up at Smith. Word for word, she repeated what had been said in the dream. The wording of the telegram too was precisely as in the dream.

Nurse Smith arrived home just in time to speak to her most loved brother before he died.

Chapter Nine

Husky and I felt all puffed up with pride when we donned our second year uniform for the first time. Now, probationers and P.T.S. students, seeing our Checks, looked at us shyly. Husk was on Wharrie, Gynaecological Ward, where, with shining eyes she was learning the mysteries of women's diseases. For me, a small miracle had happened; I was on Thistlethwayte, Male Surgical Ward, opposite Manvers, and Rene was my Staff Nurse!

The Sister was affectionately known as 'Dolly' Thistlethwayte. A most attractive woman in her mid-forties – dainty, with a waspish waist and slender ankles that were the envy of all her plump to fat companions. Iron-grey, curly hair, deep-set green eyes and impudent retroussé nose, a face vibrant with vitality. Dolly was a trotter. In fact, she out-trotted me to the extent that on her ward I was always 'on the run'.

And until they got used to her unusual routine, Sister Dolly was a terror to all her staff nurses. Rene was very nervous at first and it took her two full weeks to find the way of keeping up with Dolly's speed. When she came on duty at eight-thirty, Sister expected to find the ward scrupulously tidy, dressing trolley ready for action, the patients lying as still as mice with bandages unpinned ready for her nimble fingers to get to work.

As soon as she'd taken the night nurses' report, the 'round' started. From beds one to eighteen, she whisked from patient to patient, her butterfly fingers fluttering from trolley to wound – from wound back to trolley. Skilfully, painlessly, she changed dressings, probed wounds and removed stitches, to the accompaniment of a steady patter of commands to her harassed staff nurse, trying to keep up with her:

"Scissors, Nurse, forceps . . . Now, the probe – *quick, quick* – drop that soiled dressing in the pail – put that in the steriliser, hold this leg up, put it down . . . Oh, dear, dear, clumsy, *clumsy,* you *must* touch lightly, Nurse – *lightly.*"

And then, almost purring, she'd stop and talk soothingly to the patient:

"There now, Dad, (or Sonny) – that didn't hurt, did it? Not so bad, eh?" And to a restless one, "Lie still, lie still, my dear – much quicker if you lie still – my, but you are brave." And at times when pain was unavoidable, "Now, I'm afraid this is going to hurt, Dad, but, we'll do it ev-er so gent-ly, *ev*-er-so-*gently*," while her lovely hands worked swiftly and with incredible gentleness.

Not long after we'd been on the ward it became clear that romance was in the air. A poignant romance, for it was obvious to Rene and me that the delightful Sister Dolly was in love with a tall, handsome medical student, about twenty-six years old, and about to take his finals. Obvious too that he was as deeply in love with her. In those days hospital rules were rigid; any nurse found 'going out' with student or doctor, or even talking to either for an unnecessary length of time, risked instant dismissal. And too, sisters of wards did *not* give tea to students or doctors in the sitting-room off her ward.

The love affair was a grand passion, and Sister, sensing our unspoken sympathy occasionally took courage in both hands and entertained her beloved to tea. At such times she'd say, "Nurse dear, if anyone should come whilst I'm having tea, just tap three times on my door." We interpreted 'anyone' to mean Matron or a doctor. In this event the lover would nip up into the loft above the sitting-room until the danger had passed.

Both of us were worried about Sister's sudden and uncontrollable attacks of coughing, and often, when her cough-medicine bottle was empty, I had to fly with it down to the basement dispensary, leaving her in the kitchen gasping for breath. When I returned I'd find her limp, and purple in the face. After the medicine had eased her, she would smile her charming smile and say, "Oh, dear, Nurse – this silly old cough!"

Then, when telling us the news that her fiancé had qualified with high honours, Dolly looked truly radiant. And on the following day she handed in her resignation. She was married within a month, and tragically was dead three months later – a sudden death during a bout of coughing. The doctor was heart-broken and left London. We never heard of him again.

Dolly Thistlethwayte however, was not forgotten; sensitive nurses on night duty insisted they heard her quick footsteps trotting up and down the ward. Some went further, declaring they heard a whisper: "Nurse, Nurse! Come here . . . come quickly!"

It was during this romance that I too received an odd kind of proposal. From a youngish man who'd not spoken a dozen words since his admittance to the ward. He had a fractured spine, and was in a plaster-cast and nursed 'flat' and so in constant need of attention. My efforts at gay talk failed to coax him out of his brooding silence. He had a kind face and soulful eyes. Soon I became conscious that he was watching me up and down the ward, and as the days passed the mute appeal in his eyes, deepened.

One evening, while I was bathing him, he burst out jerkily:

"Nurse, the doctor says I can go home soon."

"Well," said I cheerfully, "that *is* good news."

He stared at me dumbly, then all in a rush, stammered:

"N-nurse, you – are -s-so- like my dead wife . . . I-I *s-swore* I'd never marry again, but you are her image . . . And, my three children need a mother . . . Nurse, *will you marry me*?"

The proposal came like a bolt from the blue. I had not read his medical notes, so did not know he was a married man. His only visitors were an elderly lady and three small children, he never spoke to us about them. The proposal was so solemnly serious I could not pass it off as a joke. So I said, just as seriously, that love was not for me, and this I firmly believed. He looked shocked as I stated firmly, in the mode of those days, "I *much* prefer platonic friendship!"

He looked at me sorrowfully, "You'll never be really happy, Nurse, until you are married and have babies . . . I am *not* going to give up hope!"

True to his word, he haunted the door-way of the hospital for weeks. I conspired with Harvey and Curly, the hall porters, and they, Curly with a twinkle in his blue eyes, and Harvey with a twirl of his elegant waxed moustache, would warn me:

"Yon hopeful's out there again, Nurse . . . better hop out the other way."

Rene, too, at that time came in for deep hero-worship – from a cat-burglar! Dick Qualls was a prisoner from Pentonville, whose sentence was due to expire before his discharge from hospital. He was a short, dapper man with close-set blue eyes, thin, bright-red lips curled up at one end under a pinched nose, a streak of black moustache added to the devil-may-care expression. Dick Qualls was full of humour and had great courage.

When he was coming round from the anaesthetic after the major operation, he flung himself about wildly calling unceasingly:

"Angel - Angel - Angel!"

Soon after his admittance he started calling Rene 'Angel' and now only she could control him. He was very quiet the week following his awful operation – for cancer of the bowels; the prognosis was grave. He endured the horribly painful dressings stoically.

He delighted in teasing us nurses, his favourite trick being to 'pinch' our scissors from our belts when we worked at his bedside. Not once did we feel his feather fingers at work. Then one day, right in the middle of Professor Pannet's teaching round, the Professor turned suddenly to Sister:

"Scissors, Sister!"

She turned to Rene standing behind her, "Scissors, Nurse!"

Rene's hand flew to her belt – no scissors!

"Sorry, Sister!" She flew over to Dick's bed with scarlet face, while the Professor fairly danced with impatience:

"Dick!" she whispered furiously, "Have *you* got my scissors?"

He looked the picture of innocence as he produced the missing scissors from under his pillow, "Well, now, Angel," said he, with his wicked grin, "that's strange – must have slipped out of your belt!"

Later, he took to boasting about his cat-burglar activities, none of the patients trusted him. But when he was allowed up he became Rene's shadow; eager to help – fetching and carrying for the patients, and cheering them up with his tall stories. When Rene turned her bewitching smile on him, saying, "Thank you, Dick", it was amazing how that rogue's face softened into an expression of sheer worship.

On the day of his discharge we felt quite sad, for there was much that was loveable about him. He didn't know how short a time he had left to indulge his incurable passion for thieving. The patients all hid their cigarettes, and most of them sat on their wallets, as he did the round of 'good-byes'.

His sparkling blue eyes were misted as he grinned at Rene, but he said cheerily:

"Bye, bye, Angel – be seeing you." He walked jauntily out of the ward.

He was back in the ward in three weeks for his check-up with Professor Pannet, and when he strolled cockily into the ward, his eyes searched eagerly for Rene:

"Sorry, Dick," I told him, "it's her day off."

The light faded from his eyes, "Oh . . ." he slumped onto the couch and stared into space.

Presently, he came over to Sister, and very politely asked if he may go into the kitchen for a glass of water. In the rush and tension, waiting for the Professor to arrive, none of us noticed that he was absent from the ward for quite a time – later, a patient told us he'd seen Dick re-entering the ward from the ward door.

Dick was the last patient to be seen, he was told not to report for another check-up – it was too late, there was nothing that could save his life. When he left the ward he called out to me:

"So long, Nurse Morris, give my love to Angel – so long."

And then, soon afterwards we discovered that two suitcases full of clothes had been stolen from the loft above the kitchen – Dick had worked quickly. The hospital had to recompense the patients for their property.

Rene was upset when I told her about it: "I know he was a thief, Ruby, but I didn't think he'd do such a mean thing, did you?"

"No, I didn't, but I bet you anything he wouldn't have thought about it if you had been on duty."

The next morning, as I was lying on my bed reading, in popped Rene, all in a rush: "Just off to change my apron, Ruby," she fished in her pocket, "got a note for you, a 'pro' from Lewis asked me to give it to you – from a patient, of all things!"

I was intrigued – who on earth would be writing me a note: I opened it quickly and read:

"Dear Nurse Morris,

Isn't it a bore! Here I am back on Lewis – pleurisy again! *Why* didn't you come and have tea with us? Cliff was so disappointed. We had arranged a chaperone, a friend, Miss Luff, and my sister, so you needn't have worried. Do please come and see us, I have never forgotten you. *Please* come.

Bill."

"Rene!" my heart was thumping with excitement, "You'll never guess who this is from . . . Remember, last year – Bill and Cliff? Well, it's from Bill!"

"There now," said Rene, eyes all aglow, "what did I tell you – it's fate. – Bill *had* to come back into your life."

"Oh, get away with you, love, you know I don't believe in fate. Your life in India has filled your head with lots of superstitious nonsense . . . Personally, I'd much rather believe I'm master of my own fate."

"One *cannot* escape destiny," returned my friend firmly, "but you're right, it is because I've lived in the East that I came to believe in fate, I've listened to many a strange tale, and *seen* so many inexplicable things."

As indeed she had. I'd listened – to tales of entranced men with skewers thrust through cheeks and arms; of tongues slashed by a razor and no flow of blood, and with quick twist of tongue, the spontaneous healing; of men sitting with one limb extended until it withered into a rock-like stick; others, who, in deep trance, entombed themselves for months, emerging at a specified date, wasted, but alive. I listened, but believed such tricks were for the gullible. I was young, sceptical, and though in many ways hypersensitive, Martha's evolving personality was daily making me more analytic and critical.

Visiting in other wards was taboo, but I knew that Nylslie Pearce was on night duty on Lewis. She would let me speak to Bill for a few minutes. By the time I went to the ward, most of the patients were asleep. "Hello, Morris," she greeted me in a whisper, "Rene told me you were coming – he's in bed eighteen, he's awake, but don't stay long, his 'temp' is high."

Bill was breathing heavily and lay back against the pillows; despite the dimmed lights, he looked more handsome than I had remembered:

"Hello, Bill," I said quietly.

He opened his eyes, and his flushed face broke into his charming smile, "Hel-*lo*, Nurse Morris – so you're still trying to make yourself into a nurse? I never thought you'd stick it!"

"Oh, I plod on . . . But never mind about me, I'm so sorry you are ill again."

"It's not too bad this time, the only thing that scares me is T.B. This is my third attack, you know."

"Oh, goodness, don't think about such a thing," said I, knowing but little about it, "you won't get it, you're far too strong . . . How's Cliff?"

"Oh, he's fine – but *why* didn't you come, were you afraid of us? I assure you we're quite harmless."

Still whispering, I lied stoutly, "Of course we weren't afraid – I lost your address . . . Are you still at the same flat?"

"Yes, we are, and once more I invite you and Nurse Drake to come over for tea – write down the address *now* – number five, St. Stephen's Road, Bayswater."

I scribbled it down hurriedly, he looked tired and very flushed, so I said: "I must go now, Bill; you do know I'm breaking a rule in coming here, don't you? I can't come again."

He pretended to pout, "I'm fed up! Why aren't you here to nurse me?"

"Cheer up, and get well quickly . . . Rene and I will look forward to seeing you both soon. A Sunday is the best day."

He was drowsy now. "O.K.", his head fell back against the high stacked pillows, and his eyes closed, "Mind you don't let us . . ." He was asleep.

I had no intention of letting him down again. By now Father's warnings had lost their sting. I told Rene about the visit, "He says he'll write to me when he's back at work, but I bet," I added ruefully, "I'll never hear from him again – serve me right, too, for being so squeamish last year!"

"You'll hear, I promise you," said Rene with conviction.

But there was no time for me to ponder the question, for just before he was transferred to a convalescent home, I was changed to Casualty. The new routine was confusing at first, I seemed to spend most of the day carrying the right things to the wrong people, which exasperated them – "No, no, Nurse – *Sister* wants that . . ." from a doctor, and "No, *no*, Nurse – that's for the doctor, don't be so stupid . . ." that from Sister.

But in spite of all the rush and the bother, I liked Casualty. It was full of excitement and drama. The patients sat on the forms in the centre of the hall, chattering away like a cluster of magpies – all about operations, pain and sudden death.

I still remember the thrill of the day that I was left in charge of the Casualty department for the first time. Sister went off for her lunch hour, and the other nurse was off duty. All puffed-up with pride I sailed round the hall beaming at the few patients already filtering in for the afternoon session, the keys in my pocket making an important jingle. I tidied up trolleys and couches, feeling a regular little Florence Nightingale – until I bumped painfully into the operating table in the Emergency Room, and gazed at it – to me it was a hideous monster . . . I ruminated anxiously . . . Would I *ever* get used to assisting Dr. Kikinnis at his minor surgery. The sight of a septic finger being opened made me feel faint, anything wrong with eyes, and teeth extractions was just as bad. His experienced eye soon saw through my tricks and excuses to disappear at such moments.

One day, as he was stitching up a head wound, he turned to me testily, "Now look here, Nurse Morris, I'm sick and tired of seeing you turn pea-green and nearly passing out on me when simple things like this have to be done."

I flushed with embarrassment. "I'm sorry, sir, I can't seem to get used to this kind of thing, seeing nails being torn off, and all this kind of thing makes me feel so sick."

"Well," he went on impatiently, "you'll just have to toughen up, Nurse; if you can't stand these small things, how are you going to stand the Theatre . . . ? There's only one way to cure you; next time a nail needs removing, *I'll* give the gas, and *you* shall do the job."

I shuddered, "I just simply could not do it, sir."

"*Cannot,* Nurse? You *will* do it – that's an order!"

The awful moment came, and while preparing the trolley, my theme song of escape echoed in my mind – I won't think about it – I won't think about it . . . just *will not* think about it . . .

And then, orders from the doctor, "Ready now, Nurse – get on with it, be quick!"

Drenched in sweat I got on with it . . . The experiment did not cure me, to this day my flesh creeps at such sights.

Two cases at that time remain vividly in my memory. Both medical. Room 7 was reserved for all medical cases – a long, narrow room containing a low bed, small table, and in the window alcove, a porcelain basin and big jug of water.

One morning, the St. John Ambulance unit brought in two women who'd collapsed in the street. The lady doctor on duty told me to prepare them for examination. She was brittle hard and full of defiance against the attitude of the male doctors, who in those days did not welcome women into the profession.

These two unfortunates left such an impression on my mind that, had I the gift, I could paint their faces today. They were sisters, the elder, plain and about thirty-five, the younger in her twenties, utterly beautiful in a 'Burne-Jones' way. Both olive-skinned, possibly foreigners. I found them huddled together in a corner of the bed, the older woman with her arms clasped protectively around her sister. They looked hunted, haunted, and were the picture of despair.

At my "Good-morning", they stared at me in silence and crouched further into the corner. Neither said a word as I prepared them for examination. "Don't be afraid," I said quietly, "No-one will hurt you, the doctor just wants to check your heart and lungs."

Empty words, I thought, "No one will hurt you" – life itself had already harmed them irreparably. The doctor was brief. After taking one quick glance at them, she looked disgusted, addressing them rather roughly.

The older woman said, "My sister and I are hungry, doctor, so hungry."

She grunted, and when she'd finished questioning them, she said:

"You're quite all right – nothing organically wrong with either of you – get dressed."

Outside the room she told me caustically, "They're prostitutes – get rid of them as soon as you can."

"But, Doctor," I protested, "they are terribly hungry – can't I give them something?"

"My *dear* little nurse, if we fed every prostitute that's brought in here, we'd never find time to do anything else . . ." she turned away, but relented and called over her shoulder, "Oh, all right, all right, give them some milk if you like."

It was the lunch hour and I was alone. I went back into the room; "Would you like some warm milk?"

"Not for me, thank you, Nurse," the elder replied, "but my sister has been so sick . . . perhaps . . ." she looked down at the young girl with such an expression of tenderness, it made my throat ache, "Will you have some milk, darling? Try some, it'll give you some strength."

The young girl spoke for the first time, her voice too, was soft, gentle and cultured, "I couldn't swallow milk, but I would love a cup of Bovril, Nurse."

"You shall certainly have it," I said, and hurried away.

For some reason Bovril in those days was as precious as gold, always kept locked in Sister's cupboard, and issued only on written instructions from a doctor.

I popped the kettle on, and unlocked the cupboard. As footsteps approached I hid the bottle of Bovril under my apron. It was the lady doctor, "Have you got rid of those women yet?"

"Soon will, Doctor, just heating some milk for them."

"Well, hurry, hurry – get rid of them as soon as possible," she snapped and rushed away.

I carried two steaming mugs to them, "Take your time." I was embarrassed at the expression on their faces.

When it was nearly time for me to go to lunch, I went back to them. "Do you feel any better? The doctor says it's not necessary for you to rest any longer."

The older woman got up. "I quite understand, Nurse," she held out her hand to her sister, "Come, darling, we must go." The girl rose and swayed a little. They looked so forlorn I could have wept. It so happened I had a half-crown in my pocket, I pressed it into the elder's hand: "Wish I had more . . . But please take your sister and get her something to eat." I turned on my heel and fled.

I had lunch in moody silence, I tried to banish their faces. At that time my knowledge of such wretchedness was about nil, but I was sure for them it was a tragedy of circumstances. And as soon as I got back to Casualty, the first person I saw was the elder sister. She came towards me slowly; I smiled at her, wondering why they had not gone. She stopped in front of me, and held out her hand, in her palm was my half-crown.

Very quietly, she said: "Nurse, my sister and I cannot take your money – you nurses get so little . . . You need it . . . For us, it cannot help . . ." she went on dully, "For us, there is only the streets . . . the streets . . ."

She walked slowly towards the door marked 'Exit'.

The following day, my eye caught sight of a small item of news in the paper . . . Two women, sisters, had been picked up in Edgware Road. They had been taken to Holloway prison, where, stated the article, they had been put in the mental department to be kept under observation . . .

Chapter Ten

One morning after lunch I got back to Casualty in time to find Nurse Nevin hurriedly emerging from Room 7, she locked the door, looking upset and frightened. I followed her to Sister's office, and when we entered it, she said defiantly:

"I *will not* stay in there alone, Sister, that woman is dangerous!"

Sister snorted, "Well, Nurse, if you've no control over the patient, there's no point in you being there . . . Ah, Nurse Morris, you're back . . . Good, I want you to go and guard the patient in seven – she's a post-epileptic mania."

I glanced at the frightened nurse, "Shall I be long in there, Sister?" I asked nervously.

"Oh, no, Nurse, the ambulance is due any moment now to take her away, but in any case," there was an ironic gleam in her eye, "I understand you're good at handling the mentally confused."

In spite of my reputation of being able to control hysterical patients, I felt anything but confident as I unlocked the door, stepped inside and locked it again, almost in one movement. I leaned against the door to assess the situation. The patient was crouching in the corner of the bed; a small, plump woman with wispy grey hair, almost colourless eyes; her face tinged with sickly pallor. She wore a dowdy costume, a tattered black hat sat askew on her head.

Having imbibed a little of the mysteries of mesmerism and psychology, I thought this an opportune moment to try out some of their theories:

"Hello, my dear," I started, in the tone of voice which infers 'God's in his heaven – all's well with the world'. "You're feeling *much* better now after your fainting spell, aren't you?"

She glared at me, at the door, then back at me again, and shouted in a horrible voice:

"Where's *she* gone to?"

"Who?" I asked innocently.

"That girl. She tried to strangle me!"

"Oh, *that* one . . . Don't worry, dear, she's not coming back, she's gone out shopping."

There was no chair in the room, so I sat on the table and tried to coax the story of her troubles from her. She crouched closer to the wall, staring at me with cunning, insane eyes. Only a few inches separated us; out of the corner of my eye I noticed I'd forgotten to fill the water-jug.

I took it as a good sign when with a sudden sob, the pathetic story burst out . . . The source of her troubles was her son, Henry, an only child and, if her story was true, he was a heartless no-good. She sniffed, and droned on and on, until eventually I was lulled into a false sense of security. Up to that moment my eyes had never left her face; she's all right now, I thought, and allowed my attention to wander. I glanced out of the window:

In a split second she leapt from the bed and grabbed the water-jug; "You slut!" she screamed, and flung up her arm to crash the jug down onto my head.

Fear caused a surge of abnormal strength in me; I caught her arm, wrenched the jug away from her, and pushed her back onto the bed, and in a voice I scarcely recognised as my own, I commanded:

"You lie down, you *stay down* – and *don't you dare move so much as a finger*."

So there we were – staring at each other, I praying the ambulance would soon come, and she starting to whimper, "I want my boy – my Henry – where is he?"

I answered more quietly, "If you behave yourself, you will be seeing your son soon." And hoped I was stating a truth.

Again I settled myself on the table. I mustered all my concentration and willed her to go to sleep. I'd already been in there half-an-hour, and when another twenty minutes went by and she was still wide awake, the strain of staring into her eyes began to tell. But she suddenly changed her tactics. She sat up on the bed, fidgeted with her clothes, then assumed a little girl expression. She cocked her head on one side like an impudent sparrow, looked at me archly, her eyes veiling some triumphant thought. Then in a thin, little voice she stated firmly:

"Want to pee!" and lowered her eyes, gazing modestly at her lap.

"Oh, dear me," said I, "that's awkward – are you *sure*?" She fluttered her eyelids at me, "Quite sure!" Her expression clearly indicated, '*Now* I've put you on the spot – what are you going to do about it?'

What indeed? There was nothing in the room to take care of the situation, neither was there a bell to ring. I dared not turn my back on her and call for help. So I decided to take a chance on it and get her to the toilets, which were at the far end of the hall. I thought my only chance was to act the 'loony' myself. I started the act by giving a silly giggle, then spun a long tale about the crowd of people outside who, poor things, were quite, quite, mad. We had to pass all these people to get to the toilet, and so we must walk very quietly, not look at them, or show any interest in them, for "You *never* know what they might do . . ." I ended.

It worked like a charm. She gave an equally silly giggle, and like a child, entered into the conspiracy:

"Right," I said, with thumping heart, "let's go."

She stood up and allowed me to straighten her clothes.

Her eyes were horrible to behold, seemingly half a dozen people lay behind them – all of them sinister.

I unlocked the door. I tucked her arm in mine and we proceeded slowly through the long hall, with heads bent close, we exchanged whispers about the poor, unfortunate 'loonies' sitting on the forms, who no doubt were intrigued by our titters and giggles. Our objective was reached without incident. I wedged myself halfway in the door – just in case.

Presently came the little girl voice: "Finished, Nurse." She emerged smiling sweetly.

All went well until I got her back in the room. As soon as I'd locked the door, she flung herself headlong onto the bed, and set up ear-splitting screams, banging her head violently against the wall. Mercifully, at that moment came a sharp rap at the door, I backed to it and unlocked it . . . two stalwart men entered, one of whom carried a strait-jacket. After a short struggle they had the poor soul secure in the jacket, and carried her away screaming 'blue murder'.

And so, trembling from head to foot and feeling as limp as a rag I went down to tea. I sat beside Nurse Rodgers, a senior nurse who had done two years training at a hospital for mental diseases. She glanced at me kindly; "Why so pale, Morris?" I told her about the patient, then added:

"Do you know, Nurse, I'm really interested in mental illness. If I manage to get through here, maybe I'll go in for it."

She looked at me keenly before replying:

"Look, Morris, I know a lot about mental nursing and I know a bit about you. Take my advice, *never* be tempted to go in for it – you are far too imaginative – you'd soon start imitating the patients, and end up a loony yourself . . . Stay away from it; study the theory if you must, but stay away from the practical."

On sober reflection I decided she was right, and thereafter retained interest in theory only.

Mondays usually started with gloomy apprehension, but the following Monday brought a change in the pattern. At breakfast Sister announced I was to go to Lilian Holland, a Women's Surgical ward of twelve beds, and the happiest in the hospital. With this good news and a letter from Bill in my pocket, I tripped along gaily to my new ward on the top floor of the hospital. I could almost hear Rene saying, 'There, what did I tell you – you see? It's fate, he *had* to come back into your life!'

We were invited to tea on Sunday. Rene was on night duty and living at Norfolk Square. She was due for two nights off at the weekend, and I intended asking for my half-day on Sunday.

Sister Eales was the most junior sister in the hospital; a petite person with warm brown eyes that held the appeal of a gazelle. She endeared herself to me at once, and for all time, by allowing me off-duty that morning, and also arranging my half-day on Sunday. I dashed over to Rene at nine-thirty:

"There," I said, all breathless, "Here it is! A letter from Bill! We're going there for tea on Sunday!"

"Oh, Ruby love, there now, what did I tell you? He had to come back into your life, you see – it's fate." She screwed up her nose and grinned happily as she read the short, friendly letter, "Umm . . . I like his writing . . . Looks determined, like him . . ."

My friend Rene has an endearing, but embarrassing habit of tripping when introduced to strangers, especially if excited or nervous. The opportunity to meet Bill came when she had to go to Lewis Lloyd to borrow an instrument. Nylslie was on duty and so she went over to speak to him. He was lying down . . . Out shot Rene's hand:

"Hello, Bill! I'm Rene . . ." and promptly tripped.

"Oh Ruby," she said relating the incident, "I felt so silly – there was I, down on my knees, looking up at him!"

"He didn't *laugh* at you?" I asked anxiously.

She chuckled, "Oh, no, he sat bolt upright in bed, and with a most comical expression and royal flourish of hand, said, 'You may rise, Nurse Drake!' I *wish* you could have seen him."

And now, here we were, bursting with excitement at the prospect of having tea with two handsome young men – the first time since coming to London. That week dragged endlessly on, until at last came Saturday. And I wakened with a very sore throat and high temperature! The Home Sister took one look at me and I was immediately banished to Sick Bay; she summoned Dr. Riley urgently, and he suspected diphtheria, so took a throat swab and ordered that I was in quarantine until the report came back from the laboratory.

And so, I was horrified when later, Rene poked her head round the door; "For heaven's sake, Rene," I croaked, "*don't* come in – Dr. Riley thinks I've got 'dip'!"

"Gosh, Ruby love, you *do* look seedy . . ." she stared hard at me, "but don't worry, I'm quite sure it's not dip – I *feel* it."

Rene too was given to feeling things:

"I'm not going to the flat without you," she added firmly.

"Oh, *Rene,*" I protested thickly, "we can't let them down again! They really will think we're afraid of them – you *must* go."

And that was why it was Rene who was the first to visit 5 St. Stephen's Road, in Bayswater. She sneaked in again to see me before setting off, looking most attractive in a neat costume, with her golden curls escaping from under a perky little hat; "Oh, Ruby, love, I just hate going alone," but her blue eyes glowed with excitement, "I feel so nervous – I'm sure to trip when I meet Cliff!"

"You're sure to if you worry about it, Rene. Do tell them how disappointed I am, and say I'll come as soon as I'm better."

As the door closed behind her I almost wept with self-pity. But that vanished when Sister came to take my temperature that evening, and told me I had not got diphtheria. But she tut-tutted anxiously on reading the thermometer: "It's still very high, Nurse," she said quietly, "But don't worry, we'll soon get rid of this fever – I'll send Nurse Smith in to give you a tepid-sponge."

I felt more comfortable after the bath, and now I knew I had not got diphtheria I was in a fever of impatience to see Rene, who insisted she would come in to see me before going to bed. It was ten thirty when she came, by which time my temperature was again soaring. One look at her face told me the day had been a success; she glowed with enthusiasm. "Oh, I've had a wonderful, wonderful day . . . they . . ." she stopped short as she glanced at my chart, "Heavens, your 'temp' is a hundred and four! You must be feeling ghastly – I'll tell you all about it tomorrow."

"You'll do no such thing, Nurse Drake," I said with muffled firmness, "the day's been an eternity . . . You just sit down over there and tell me *everything* . . . But before you start you'll be glad to know you were right, I've not got 'dip'."

"Thank goodness for that, but honestly, Ruby, I shouldn't stay – if I'm caught Sister will report me to Matron."

"You won't be, Rene, Sister and the Charge-nurse came at ten." I settled myself against the damp pillows, "Now . . . Begin . . ."

While she talked on I closed my burning eyes and conjured up vivid pictures of the day's happenings. Her description of Cliff was exactly as I'd imagined:

"He's absolutely charming, Ruby," she went on dreamily, "Not as tall as Bill, very slender, tremendously good looking. It was he who opened the door, then Bill came running down the stairs. He looked very disappointed seeing me alone, but was quick to hide it. He gave that lovely smile of his, and said, 'Oh, what a shame, I'm so sorry she's sick. But please, do go on up'."

"Did you feel shy?"

"No, I didn't . . . Imagine *me* not being shy! But they're so natural I felt at home immediately."

"Thought they'd be like that," I murmured.

"I don't know if he's always like that," Rene went on, "but I just can't imagine Cliff ever being depressed. He seems just bubbling over with the sheer joy of being alive. His eyes are greenish-hazel, and he has the most *lovely* speaking voice."

I tried to ignore my splitting head. "Go on, Rene, describe the flat . . ."

After she had gone, pictures of the day that I had missed, the day I had so looked forward to – floated before my inner vision . . . I saw Rene arriving at the old Georgian house that had known better days; watched her climb the three long flights of stairs, and stop at the end of the landing in front of the blue door with a brass knocker.

The four-roomed flat was bright and shining, looking greatly cherished. In the neat, spotless kitchen, a canary chirped a cheery welcome as he hopped around his cage. The sitting-room had a distinct atmosphere of its own; artistically arranged, fragrant with flowers beautifully arranged in decorative vases. Flame-coloured drapes covered the window which overlooked the road, the curtains were drawn against the gloom of the November afternoon. Bookshelves at the left of the window were packed with books, titles mostly of poems, plays, and essays, together with some good novels. On the other side of the window was a large gramophone cabinet; opposite the window against the wall, a dark-oak sideboard held a vase of flowers and a few oriental ornaments.

On either side of the gas fireplace a comfortable armchair, above the mantelpiece an oval mirror, in which reflected the oval gilt-framed picture of the 'Mona Lisa' on the opposite wall. A brown carpet, shaded table lights, one or two straight-backed chairs; a humpty, gate-legged table and a small round table completed the picture of the room – a room designed to shut out the hustle and bustle of city life.

I turned over feverishly, and the visions merged into crazy patterns – weaving carpet, fallen roses, books upside down, flickering lights, and Mona Lisa smiling down enigmatically onto the flower-scented room.

Suddenly, I slept.

Chapter Eleven

Four weeks later, Rene and I jumped onto a Bayswater bus. This time it was I who felt shy. Rene laughed as she tucked her arm in mine.

"You won't feel shy for long, I promise you."

It was Bill who opened the door; "At last, at long last," he smiled warmly, "Nurse Morris, I'm very happy to welcome you to our home."

As we went up the stairs, Cliff popped his head round the kitchen door; "Hel-*lo,* Nurse Morris! I really began to think you were a myth."

We all shook hands.

It was just as Rene had said, Cliff seemed buoyant with optimism. He darted back into the kitchen, and started whistling to the canary.

The flowers looked lovely:

"That's Cliff's job," said Bill, "he does the flowers and puts all the 'spit and polish' on the flat – I do the cooking."

"Well," said I, in rapt admiration, "it certainly works well – it's all so lovely."

He drew the curtains and switched on the shaded lights; and with the warmth from the gas-fire and the room's soft, orange-blue tints, it was hard to believe that outside it was cold and damp.

"Excuse me for a moment," said our host, "I'll just help Cliff get tea."

From the depth of the arm-chair I suddenly felt drowsy. I remembered the crazy upside-down pictures, and the clear pattern of the room that had appeared when I was wracked by fever . . . I closed my eyes, then just as suddenly, opened them and sat up . . . I looked straight into Mona Lisa's eyes. She looked down at me with inscrutable expression, and it gave me the shivery impression that the room was – waiting. Impatiently, I shrugged the feeling away.

It was impossible to feel shy for long in the presence of these two cheerful young men. Bill's home-made cakes were delicious. They kept up amusing chatter, and when we had finished tea, Cliff remarked in the most natural way: "Look, we can't go *on* calling you by your surnames, can we?" So Christian names were adopted, but Cliff always called me 'Rube'.

That Sunday afternoon set a seal on a delightful and I suppose, unique friendship – a friendship that lives to this day. Throughout that winter, and on into the spring, our relationship with Bill and Cliff blossomed into serene mutual understanding, and save for occasional visits, Lyon's Corner House dropped out of our world.

Instead of listening to 'syrupy' music, we heard the music of the masters – carefully chosen records, excerpts from the operas; Galli-Curci, Fritz Kreisler, John MacCormack, Tchaikovsky and Chopin were among our favourites. We were young and in love with life, these sessions transported us to another world – a world whose major hero was John Keats.

An evening came when Bill, in a very masterful way, said: "Now, look here, Ruby Morris, Cliff and I have been waiting for weeks to hear you sing . . . No more excuses this evening if you please – over you go to the door. You needn't feel shy, we won't look at you, I'll put the light out."

I'd excused myself on account of there being no piano, afraid of pitching a song too high and cracking on a top note. But that evening I was full of the 'hwyl' and obeyed without a word of protest. Fortunately the pitch was true and the high notes came forth without disaster. I ended the 'recital' with nostalgic Welsh ballads, then sat down. Not a word was uttered for a long moment, and I went fiery hot with embarrassment, thinking I must have sounded tinny or out of tune.

Then Bill said quietly, "Well, Ruby dear, what you are doing in a hospital when you possess a voice like that I simply cannot imagine."

"That's what I feel too," said Rene.

Cliff echoed, "It's a crime – it really is!"

"I'm in a hospital, Bill, for the same reason that you work in a big London store – family circumstances. We all have to earn our living."

"But," Bill came back eagerly, "I have friends in the theatre, I can get you auditions – I'm *sure* I can get you on the stage."

"No, Bill," I said firmly, but with regret, "it's too late – I am determined to qualify as a nurse."

There was a sharp contrast between hospital routine and our off-duty times; we lived in two entirely different worlds. As time went on our love for literature deepened, and also the passion for music and the arts in general. Particularly lovely were the sessions of poetry reading. Usually they were read by Bill whose well-modulated, musical voice carried us along on wings of delight; especially his favourite poem 'The Ode To A Nightingale', which he often recited after an evening of listening to records.

Then too, at times like these, Bill – with shattering change of mood, rather like a Welsh preacher descending from a high note of the 'hwyl' – would lapse into such a spate of hilarious cockney humour, that in seconds he would have us tumbling down from the clouds, helpless with laughter. And so, he always maintained a balance between the sublime and the ridiculous. We four had very little money to spend but that didn't stop us from having blissfully happy times together. Rene and I saved as many pennies as we could, and when possible we four picnicked in the country – Shenley Wood being the most favourite spot. And we often managed to take flowers to the flat.

And so, in the early spring of 1926, the flat at 5 St. Stephen's Road became the focal point of what the four of us considered a fine human relationship. Due no doubt to our Victorian upbringing – and in my case to Father's fearful warnings – Rene and I took refuge in the world of 'platonic' ideals, and in that world we were determined to stay. Hazy but earnest ideas of philosophy, love and religion were exchanged with great seriousness; but the stresses of hospital life and the work-a-day world were strictly taboo. Thus steeped in verse and music we escaped from reality.

Often too our number increased to include Bill's mother, a great character with a never-failing sense of humour, his sister, a tall, striking young woman, and other friends. Cliff's parents lived at Lowestoft.

We wanted so much to include Husky in this companionship, and Bill and Cliff went on patiently repeating their invitation to come and join us. But Husky, being the ardent, dedicated nurse did not at first approve of the friendship, and maintained that I, in particular could not afford to take my mind off medical things, and waste time in gathering what she insisted was a lot of woolly ideas:

"What about your exams, Ruby? You should be studying," she would reprimand me.

And I'd insist that I was able to study much better by getting the complete break from hospital routine.

"Well, it's your lookout."

But bit by bit I wore her down, and eventually she weakened and said she'd come, "But not until our exams are over!"

Examinations! Once again the bugbear of my life was looming depressingly close. Although I stoutly declared studying was easier after sessions at the flat, I knew in my heart it was not true. For while trying to take in medical and surgical knowledge, I'd find my mind wandering and pondering on the beauty of friendship.

But now I realised that friendship must be put on one side, and both Bill and Cliff understood when I told them that I could not come again until the exams were over. And so I settled down to intensive study in my off-duty times. The weeks sped by in a frenzy of swotting through books, and never-ceasing questions:

"What does so and so mean, Husky?"

"Why does it happen? How is it treated?"

"How on earth do you pronounce this ghastly word, Rene?"

On and on, until at last the dreaded week arrived, which I faced with acute apprehension, suffering the usual vomiting attacks. I also had to re-sit my first year medical paper.

With the nightmare over, Husky and I anxiously scanned the list of names posted on the notice-board. The print became a blur, for I could not see my name anywhere . . . Husky caught my arm as I swayed:

"It's all right, Ruby, it's all right – you've passed them all. Your marks are a bit low, but you've passed, love, you've passed!"

My eyes focused. There was Husky – right at the top of the list, and there was I – right at the bottom.

Examination week coincided with pay day – between us Rene and I had six pounds! So on our next half-day we scuttled about and bought a chicken, a bottle of white wine and a dozen roses . . . It was Husky's evening off and she was coming to the flat for the celebration dinner, given in honour of her splendid results, and Martha's humble victory. It was a gay, light-hearted evening. Bill in one of his ridiculous moods, kept us all in fits of laughter. Husk was very impressed and en route back to hospital, remarked: "Goodness, Ruby, are they always like that? I haven't laughed so much for years!"

"Oh, dear me, *no*, usually we're terribly serious – discussing world problems and poverty, or reading poetry and plays, and listening to records."

My friend grinned impishly, "Wouldn't appeal to me, I like only nonsense rhymes in the way of poems."

And of these she had a large repertoire, and often to try and snatch me out of the 'blues', she'd strike a comic attitude with eyes raised to heaven, and recite the one I disliked the most:

"Oh, Mama dear, what is that there
That looks like strawberry jam?
Hush, hush, my child, it's Papa
Run over by a tram."

It made me furious but had the desired effect. Husky was always on the alert to protect me, and I, to protect Rene, who was regarded as an angel by all.

It was in the month of the lilacs that my dream came true and I was able to take Rene to my home in Prestatyn, where she endeared herself even more firmly to me by falling in love with my family, and with Wales. She met George and Muriel, and their new-born twins, and they; Father, Gret and Lilas fell in love with Rene.

Then on our return from our holiday I had the shock of being sent to the theatre. Now, I murmured within myself at the breakfast table – *that* will fix you . . . I'll never be able to stick it, never! While thinking this change would be my swan-song to a nursing career, my mind went back to an awful afternoon on my third ward. I was a raw probationer of scarcely six months, and anxiously carrying out instructions, preparing a patient who was due at the theatre at two o'clock for a major operation.

All was going well, the patient was decked out in the operation gown and long woollen stockings, I'd even remembered to ask the important, "Have you got false teeth?", when along came Sister. Obviously in a benign mood, she ran her professional eye over the patient, glancing approvingly at the dentures in the tumbler:

"Very good, Nurse, very good – you haven't forgotten anything." She turned, then paused, as a sudden thought struck her:

"Nurse Morris, have you taken a patient to the theatre yet?"

"No, Sister."

"Nor seen an operation?"

"No, Sister." My heart started thumping so loudly I was sure she'd hear it.

"Well, Nurse," Sister went on pleasantly, as though giving me a treat to the movies, "as we're so quiet on the ward this afternoon, you may take the patient to the theatre. Stay by her until she is under the anaesthetic, then ask Sister Theatre for permission to go up into the gallery – tell her I would like you to have this opportunity of seeing an operation."

"Yes, Sister," said I.

"And Nurse," she went on sternly, "be sure to sit near the door. If you feel the slightest bit queer, come out *immediately* – don't you *dare* cause a commotion by fainting."

"I understand, Sister." I breathed a sigh of relief. All I had to do was to feel 'queer' and come out!

Even so, my heart raced with panic when the porter wheeled in the trolley. The patient, a gentle little soul was a little drowsy, after her injection. En route to the theatre I looked down at her quiet face, hoping to gain courage. In the anaesthetic room I called on Martha as the anaesthetist strode into the room. I took hold of the patient's hands, she looked up at me and smiled:

"Don't be afraid, Nurse dear, I shall be all right."

Watching her, I felt as though I was suffocating.

Then Sister Theatre came in through the swing doors, looking very agitated. It was Mr. FitzWilliams' operating day. He was an enormous man, six feet four inches tall, his huge hands performed operations of miraculous delicacy on tiny babies with hare-lips and cleft-palates, which were his specialities.

Just as I opened my mouth to give Sister Theatre the message about my going up to the gallery, she snapped out an order:

"Come along in here, Nurse . . . Get a cap and gown . . . Hurry, hurry . . ."

I felt riveted to the floor. "Cap and gown, Sister? W-what for?"

"Don't stand there, girl, wasting time with stupid questions – I need you in there with me – we're short of a nurse."

"You m-mean me," I gasped, "In the *theatre*?"

"Of course – where else? Don't be so silly, Nurse."

"B-but, S-sister said I was to go into the gallery . . . A-and if f-felt q-queer- I-was-to-come-out-i-immediately . . ."

She snorted impatiently, "I can't help *what* your Ward Sister told you – I have to have another nurse." She gave me a sharp push into the theatre and handed me a cap and gown.

The patient was on the table; a nurse was helping the surgeon into his gown. Privileged students stood nearby, masked and gowned, waiting to gather round the surgeon to watch the operation. Intense silence reigned; the audience in the gallery looked down on a scene that to me looked like a gathering of the Ku Klux Klan.

Sister whispered, "Stand by me, I'll tell you what to do."

But Mr. FitzWilliams had other ideas.

"Come here, little nurse," he said, peering at me over his mask, "Hold this patient's arm back."

My heart was pounding against my ribs, a mist swam before my eyes. I walked forward and took hold of the arm:

"No, no, Nurse," said the surgeon, "Further back and up . . . Yes, that's right . . . Now, hold it there."

There I stood commanding Martha to stop me from fainting, which would disgrace me for ever, but worse, might harm the patient.

Fortunately, a tall medical student whom I recognised as my ward 'dresser' moved closer to me, smiled down at me encouragingly, and placed himself in a position that shielded me from the sight of the first frightful incision. I hid behind his broad back until my guardian Martha was in complete control, then I looked, and having looked, my eyes stared hypnotically in awful fascination until the operation was over.

And with that vision foremost in mind, I tramped miserably up the stairs to the theatre, prepared for the worst. But my gloom vanished when I discovered that most operations were performed on only small areas of exposed flesh. Being the junior I hovered in the background fetching and carrying, emptying receptacles, disposing of soiled dressings and cleaning up afterwards.

My brother George was right. Here was enough drama to last a lifetime. I soon got used to theatre routine, and in time came to love the work.

Soon after being sent to the theatre, another kind of drama developed. With our friends, Bill and Cliff at the flat, Rene and I drifted innocently and casually into a series of strange happenings that for Bill and myself almost ended in complete disaster.

Chapter Twelve

It all began on the evening that Cliff came back from a weekend at his parents' home in Lowestoft. He was eager to tell us all about a party he'd been to, at the home of an elderly couple, friends of his parents. They were grief-stricken at the recent death of their son, an only child. It was a social evening among a few close friends. At midnight the bereaved parents turned to a middle-aged man,

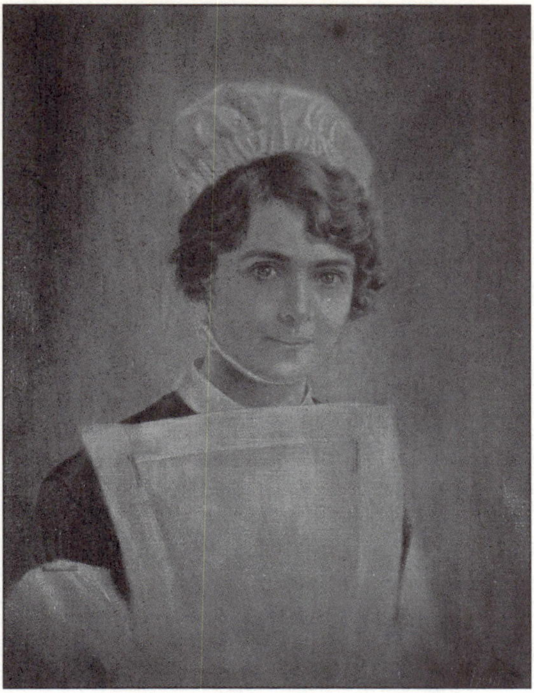

Sister 'Dolly' Thistlethwayte.
Photograph by David G. Lewis.

St. Mary's Hospital.

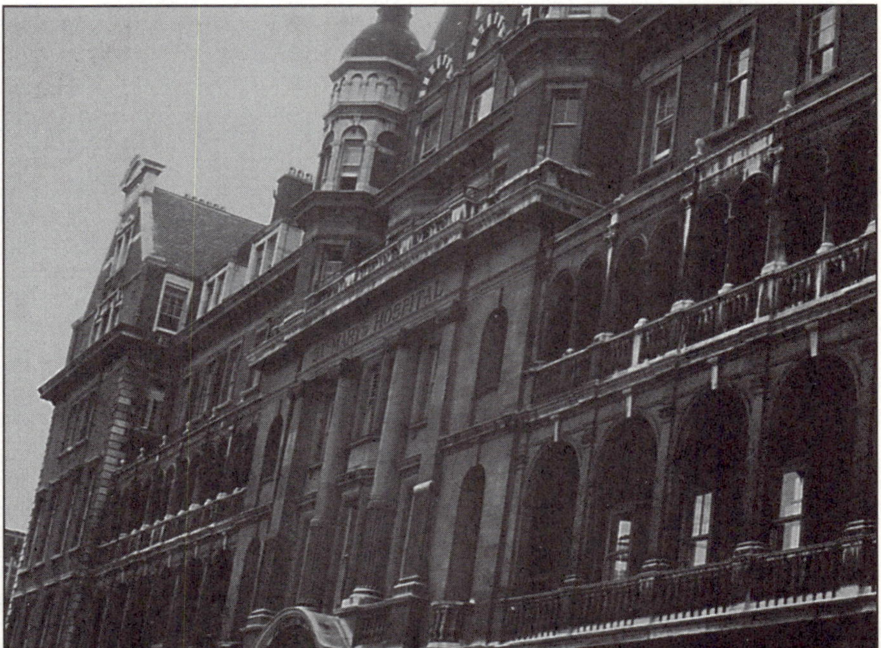

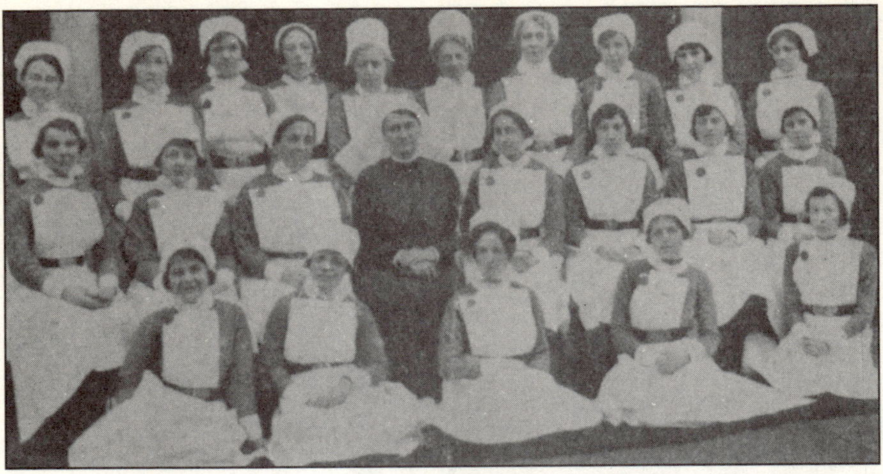

The Matron of St. Mary's surrounded by a group of her Sisters.

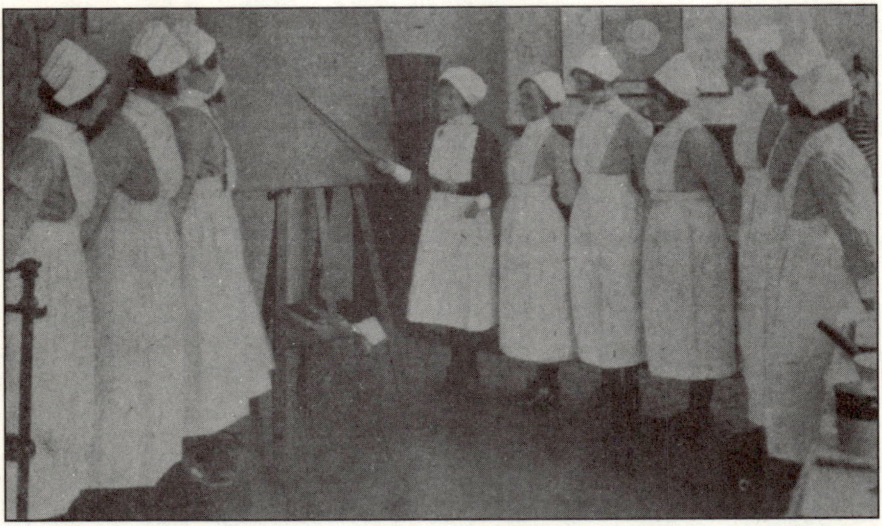

Nurses receiving a lesson in the Preliminary Training School, prior to their actual work in the wards.

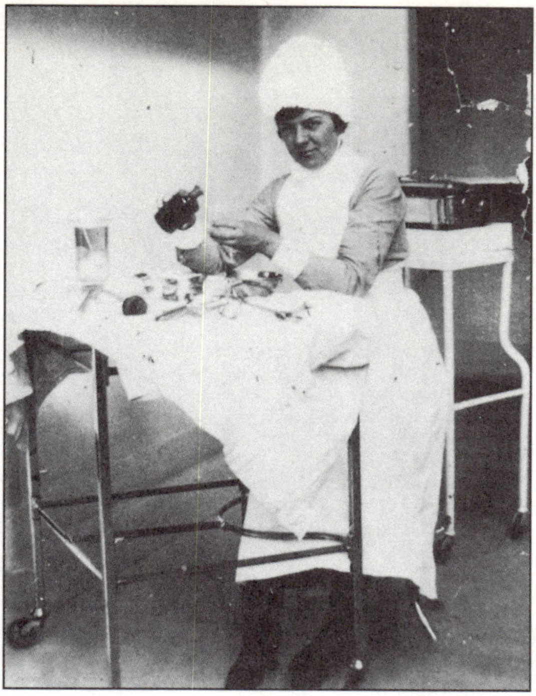

Ruby Morris in St. Mary's Theatre.

Sister with a new school of probationers.

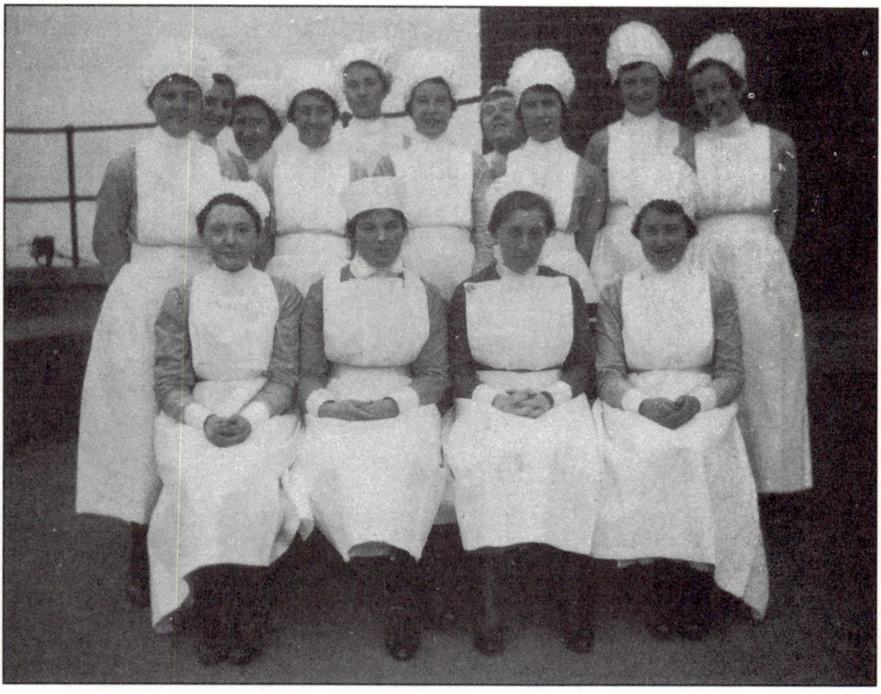

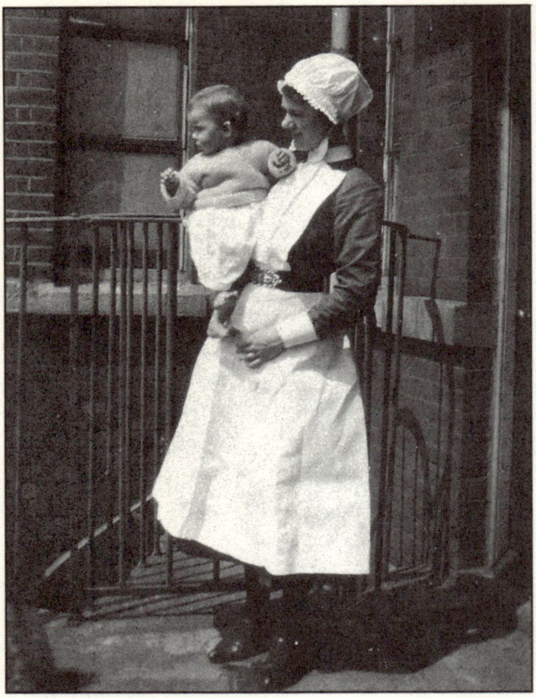

Nurse M. J. Gatward, charge nurse, the maternity ward in 1931.

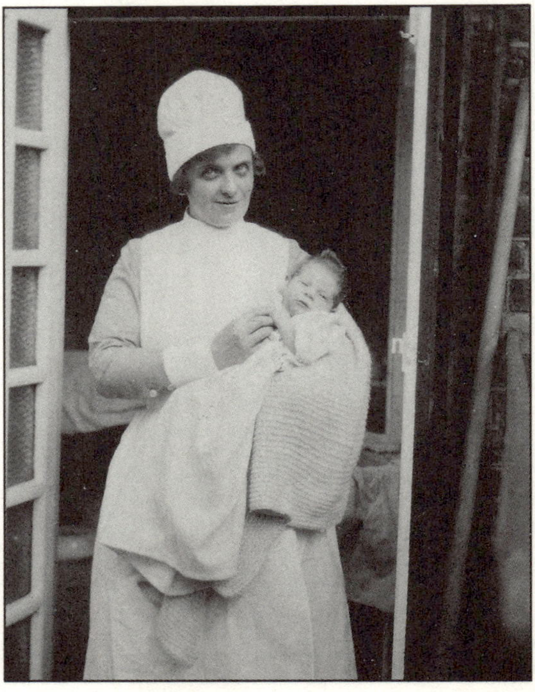

Sister in the maternity ward, 1930.

The author in Foochow, 1938, at the Kushan Monastery.

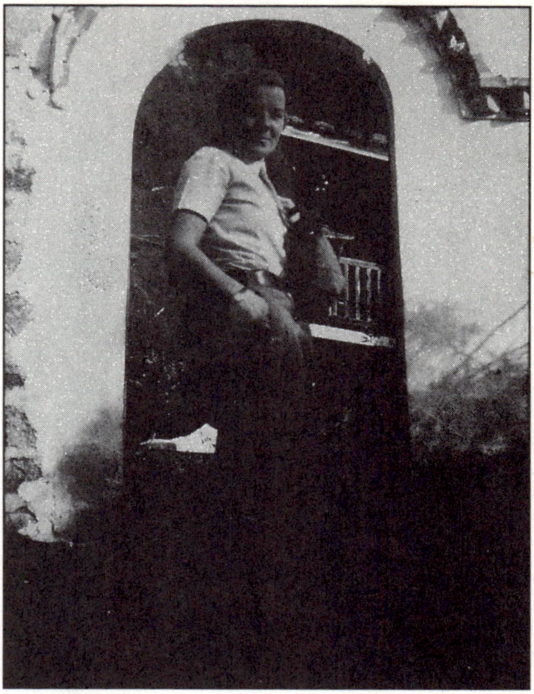

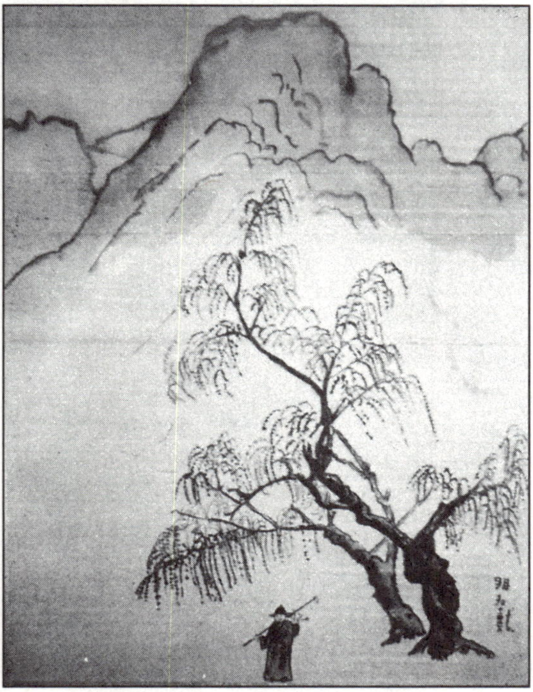

A painting on silk by Dr. Dymond, the author's husband.

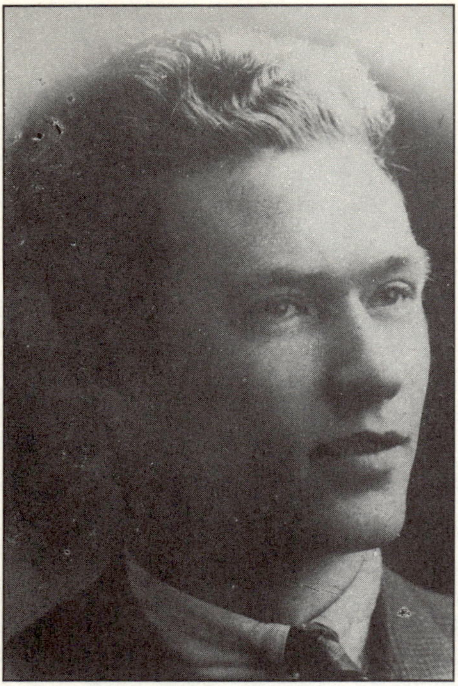

E. C. Dymond, aged 20.

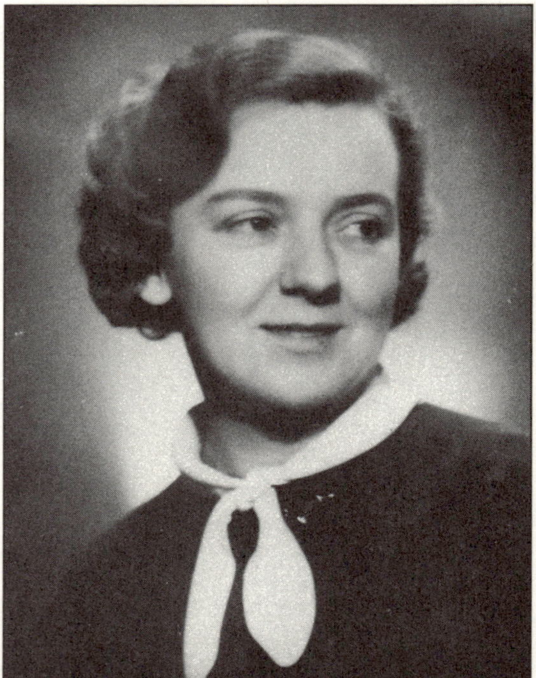

The author, aged 35, taken in Shanghai.

Nurse Irene Drake.

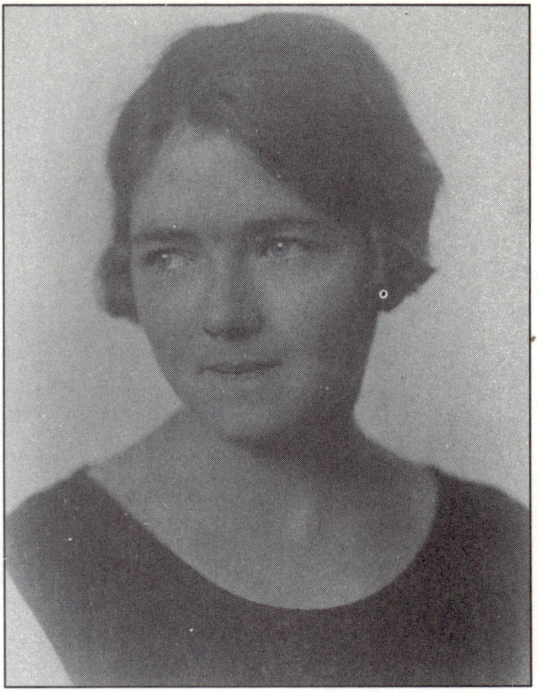

Bill Peacock, Irene Drake and Ruby Morris, 1926.

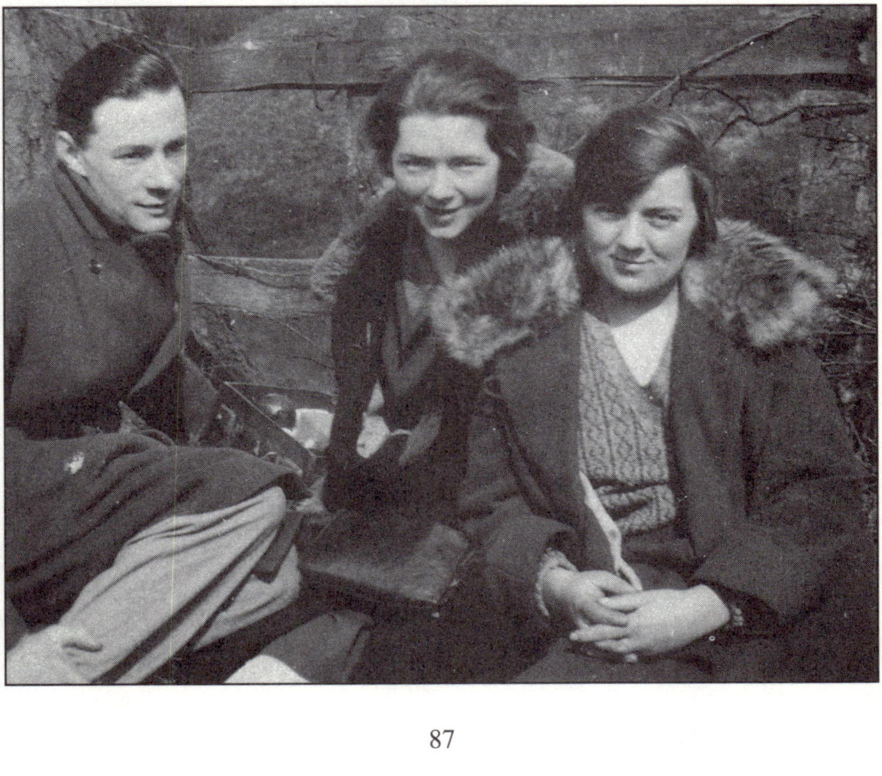

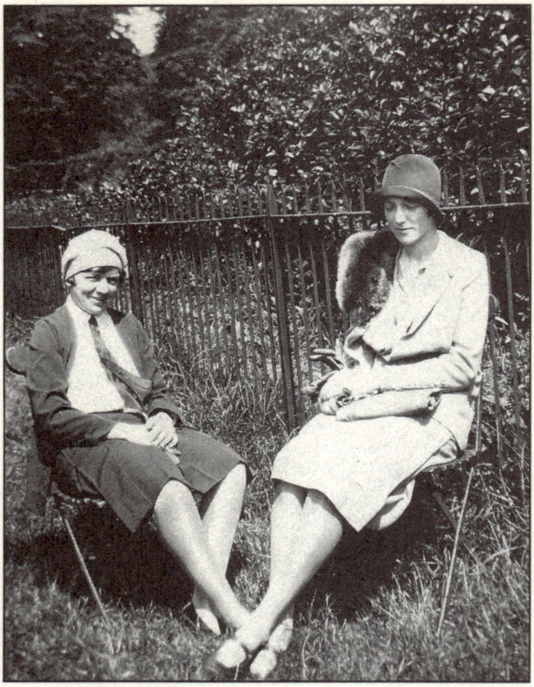

Husky and Ruby, 1926.

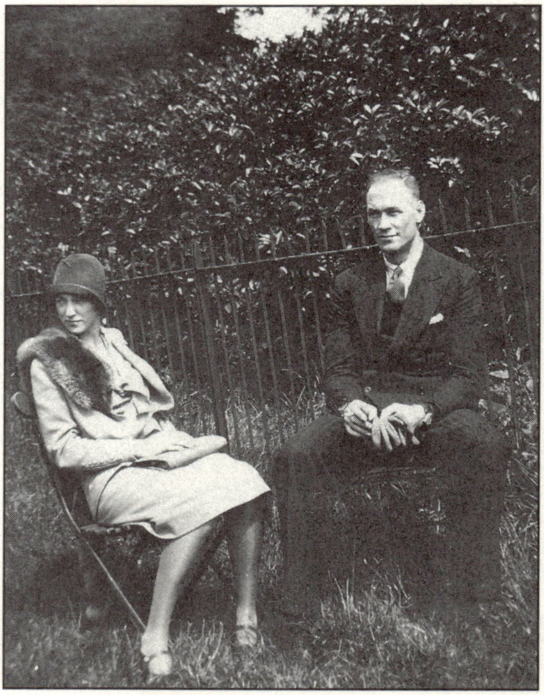

Jimmy Dymond and Nurse Huskinson.

pleading, "Please – let's try again!"

The man went and quietly brought a round table to the centre of the room: "What's all this?" Cliff wanted to know.

Someone whispered, "Table-turning, they're trying to get into touch with their son."

Listening to Cliff relating the events my curiosity was aroused:

"But Cliff . . . I don't understand . . . Table-turning! What is it exactly? I've never heard of such a thing . . . What do they do?"

He lowered his voice to a mysterious whisper. "Rube, it means getting in touch with spooks . . . spirits!"

"Pooh," chipped in Bill impatiently, "it's a lot of nonsense – don't believe a word of it."

"Don't believe a word of what, Bill?" asked Rene.

"Spiritualism!" he said, with great scorn, "They claim to have made contact with the dead, through the medium of a table or ouija board – the spirits rap out messages, so they say – absolute bilge, of course."

"Hmm . . ." Cliff broke in, "I'm not so sure, Bill, I thought it was a joke at first, or some kind of game. I watched their hands and feet thinking someone was slyly pushing the table."

"You can bet your life they were," grunted Bill.

"Well, if they were they were mighty cunning about it. They were all so terribly serious too. I didn't believe it of course, but all the same I felt nervous."

"Why, Cliff?" I queried.

"It was the atmosphere I suppose – the lights out and the eerie shadows in the room from the fire. Five of them sat round the table and joined hands. After a few minutes the table started swaying and the leader asked who was there. He spoke out the alphabet and the table stopped dead at certain letters. Then I became interested and put my hand on the table . . . I got a shock I can tell you. My fingers tingled and turned icy cold . . . I leapt back, and put on the lights. They were furious with me – said I'd broken the circuit or something."

Bill, a person of very decided views and unshakeable convictions, laughed scornfully, "*Really,* Cliff, do be your age . . . Fancy falling for bilge like that. The whole thing's phoney, those people are 'nuts'."

"Do you know any Spiritualists, Bill?" I asked.

"Great Scott, no!"

"Have you ever tried it yourself?"

"Of *course* not, it would bore me to death."

"Then," I went on, "how can you know it's nonsense?"

"Because, my dear Ruby," he came back, with dramatic flourish of hands, "I believe when one is dead, one is DEAD, and that's the end of it – finish – oblivion!"

"Well, I *don't*," I said firmly.

"What makes you so sure?" asked Cliff.

"I don't really know, possibly because of the strange feelings I get when people are dying "

"Oh, dear, there you go again," Bill started teasingly, "it's that Celtic imagination of yours . . . you're too impressionable."

I got up and fidgeted round the room, irritated at the recurring accusation; "Maybe I am too impressionable, Bill, but I *do* believe in life after death . . . In fact I'm not at all sure I believe in death at all . . . I think . . . only in change. After all, once safely born, we know we are bound to die . . . Surely it too must be part of the pattern?"

"My dear girl," Bill retorted impatiently, "why on earth should we bother our heads about such questions . . . We're young, healthy, let's stay that way. Time enough when we're old to bother about such things."

But for me, the questions: "Who am I?" "Where did I come from?" and "Where to next?" had plagued my mind from an early age. The mysterious heavens intrigued me and, also, who were the 'people' of my childhood . . . Imagination, or . . .?

And so, now, for the first time I pondered on this possibility – communion with the dead . . . But, communion through the medium of a table! Seemed to me absurd, undignified, repulsive.

I turned to Cliff to ask further questions, but Rene leapt to her feet:

"Gosh, Ruby, it's half-past nine – we must fly!"

We had no late pass so had to be in by ten.

We flung on our coats, bade our friends a hasty good-night, and fled to catch the bus.

On the way back to hospital, we remained silent and thoughtful for a time, then Rene voiced what I was thinking, "I wonder if anything would happen if we four sat round that little table?"

"Who knows – but I'm sure Bill wouldn't let us, but in any case I should think one must *believe* in it to make it happen – and we don't."

The seeds of curiosity had been planted and, until our next visit to the flat I pondered on the possibility of such contact with the dead – how exciting to investigate their origin and purpose. This flow of thought produced an evening session with Bill and Cliff on our next evening off that led us into the deep waters of serious talk about the inequalities of life, and the unequal distribution of worldly goods. Bill held powerful, sympathetic convictions about the underprivileged and minority groups. Both of them seldom missed an opportunity to help a lame dog over a stile, and in the doing, often got let down. But it did not seem to shake their faith in human nature – excuses would be found for ungrateful behaviour, and soon forgotten.

Later, over coffee and sandwiches, I found my eyes being drawn to the three-legged table in the corner, it supported a bowl of marguerites. Presently Bill said: "Whatever's the matter with you tonight, Ruby, why do you keep on staring at that table?"

"I was just wondering if we put our hands on it, whether it would move?"

There was an edge to his voice in reply, "*Whatever* made you think that?"

"I've thought of little else since Cliff talked about it."

Bill said no more, but got up abruptly and went over to the gramophone, and put on Tchaikovsky's 'Andante Cantabile'. I sat back in my chair and closed my eyes, and in a few moments, as often before, the back of my hands turned strangely cold – it felt as though a chill wind was playing on them. The weird melody crept over me and heightened the sense of awareness I so often experienced at the bedside of a dying person. I wondered if we four were the only persons in the room.

There were soft shadows around us, cast by the table-lamps and the gas-fire. When the last note of the music died away Bill opened his eyes and looked directly into mine:

"The Cantabile always has a strange effect on me," I murmured.

"Me too," said Bill as he got up and closed the cabinet, "*No more music* . . ." He sat down again, and I asked quietly:

"Bill, Rene and I really would like to try the table . . . Let's do it, just once . . . *Please*."

He moved restlessly and looked as though the reply would be a firm "No", but instead, he shrugged resignedly and said in heavy, paternal tones, "Oh, well, if you children *must* play."

"No, Bill," Cliff interrupted quickly, "I don't think we should, it really is quite uncanny, you know."

"Don't you worry, Cliff, I guarantee nothing will happen, it's all a lot of bosh; but maybe the girls will be satisfied if we try it once."

We moved the table to the centre of the room and Cliff brought in two more chairs from the back room. Rene looked excited as Cliff put out the lights – only the fire-glow remained. I silently called on Martha to remain, cool, calm and critical. We bent our heads and Cliff murmured flippantly, "We must concentrate, you know."

This is meant to be an experiment, I thought, so we should give 'them' the benefit of the doubt; so I said mentally, "If anyone is in this room, please move the table – Go on, if you're here, prove it."

Then came that strange, cold sensation in my hands, my fingers tingled . . . Suddenly, the table tilted onto one leg, then dropped as suddenly – just once. Then Bill spoke out, "I don't believe for one moment that anyone is here, but if there is, please spell out your name."

The response was immediate: A name was spelt out which meant nothing to any of us.

Some impulse made me say, "Now, look here, I do *not* believe in Spiritualism, and using a table is never going to convince me . . . Is it possible for you to use one of us instead?"

A sharp tap affirmed, "Yes."

Fascinated, I went on, "Then please move the table towards which one of us you can use."

Immediately it swayed over to Bill, then stopped:

"What must we do?" I asked.

"DIE . . . DIE . . . DIE . . ."

This sounded so melodramatic I enquired derisively, "What do you mean – DIE – do you mean mentally, or what?"

And at that moment Bill gave a sharp gasp, slumped over onto the table – apparently completely unconscious. It was so sudden and unexpected we three froze with terror:

Cliff grabbed my arm, "Rube, for God's sake *do* something!"

I was just as shocked and had no idea what to do, but intuition warned me, "Keep quiet, Cliff . . . we mustn't do anything . . . just watch."

The room was uncannily still:

In a few moments Bill drew a long, quiet breath and slowly straightened up . . . and as we looked at him we almost gasped for his face was that of a complete stranger. It must have been an illusion, but to me it seemed his face had altered in shape. Another deep breath, then he stretched his arms with a grand gesture, his eyes still tightly shut, and slowly got up.

There was no illusion about his voice, for when he spoke it was that of an old man . . . For about twenty minutes he moved about the room seemingly having a conversation between an old man and a child.

We sat there staring at him in fascinated horror, unable to move. Then Cliff made a sudden movement which knocked something to the floor.

And at the sound of it Bill gave a short gasp and fell to the floor as though pole-axed. Rene leapt to her feet and put on the lights. Cliff cried out excitedly:

"*Do* something, Rube, do something . . . bring him round!"

We lifted him up onto the arm-chair:

"Don't panic, Cliff, don't panic – he'll be all right," I assured him with more confidence than I felt."

Cliff took his friend's arm and shook it gently, "Bill, wake up, please wake up!"

Then to our intense relief, he suddenly opened his eyes, and shivered, "Oh, I am so terribly cold!"

I turned the gas-fire up, and Rene went out to the kitchen to heat some milk:

"I feel so stiff," he remarked wonderingly, and when Rene handed him the glass of hot milk and brandy, he looked surprised. "What's this for?" he asked suspiciously:

"You said you felt cold, so I got you a warm drink," said Rene soothingly.

He looked bewildered as he sipped it. Presently, he stared at us in turn, "Whatever is the matter with you three . . . why are you looking so peculiar . . . What's happened?"

Cliff looked at me appealingly.

"Come on," Bill demanded irritably, "for heaven's sake stop being so mysterious . . . Tell me!"

"Well, Bill," Cliff began hesitantly, "as a matter of fact, I-I'm afraid you went into a trance."

Bill looked dumbfounded, "Into-a-what!"

"It's true, Bill, you were in a trance for about twenty minutes."

"*Me* . . . in a trance! Don't be so absolutely absurd, Cliff, how could *I* go into a trance – I don't believe in all that bilge."

We remained silent:

"Ruby, tell me the truth . . . *Did* I go into a trance, or is this some silly joke?"

"It's no joke, Bill, you really did."

He looked horrified, "What did I do?"

We told him.

Then he looked hard at each one of us, and said with determination:

"Well, that's the first and last time you'll ever get me to put my hands on a table."

And that was the *beginning* of a strange series of happenings.

Chapter Thirteen

During my hours in the theatre cleaning up after operations, washing rubber sheets, cleaning trolley-castors, my mind tossed up various theories as to why Bill, of all people, had gone into a trance. I tried to reject the theory of 'spirits', but the possibility fascinated me. I wanted to prove it, one way or the other. 'A little knowledge is a dangerous thing', that I knew, but Martha in a muddle of 'half-baked' ideas gradually evolved a neat little theory – the table, I concluded, was moved by personal magnetism, and Bill, being an emotional person got worked up, hypnotised himself, and so fell into a trance.

From conversations of senior nurses I had learned that there was a thing called the sub-conscious mind, but how it worked I hadn't the faintest idea. But the ever analytical Martha went on probing, and one bright morning seated on the floor polishing the trolley-castors I had a sudden triumphant thought – Well, that's settled it . . . *That's* what it was, his sub-conscious mind! The four of us are emotional, dramatic; and Bill and I frustrated actors . . . The music, the dim light, we got worked up – That's it, self-hypnotism and the sub-conscious.

I wanted urgently to confirm this conclusion but I had no money to buy books on mesmerism and allied subjects, but even if I'd had the money I would not have known what to look for. I browsed in the nurses' medical library and came across an ancient, moth-eaten tome by Mesmer, not one word of which I could understand.

I talked my idea over with Rene, who shook her head doubtfully: "You may be right, Ruby, but I can't help feeling there's more to it than that. Isn't it fascinating? I *do* wish we could know for sure."

"Well, we're not likely to, I can't see Bill changing his mind, can you? I don't think we should try to persuade him."

Soon after, I was unexpectedly sent on night duty again to replace a sick nurse. I was upset at leaving the theatre as I had come to love it. And after three weeks on nights I became very restless. Rene was due for a day off, and as it coincided with a public holiday, she, Bill and Cliff had planned to go to Shenley Woods for a picnic.

The day dawned fair and beautiful, not a cloud in the sky, and only the merest hint of autumn in the air. I came off duty feeling rebellious; Rene was in my room when I got over to Norfolk Square: she greeted me gaily, "Oh, Ruby love, isn't it a glorious day . . . I *do* wish you could be with us!"

An imp of recklessness struck me – Martha's warning was banished:

"That's just what I'm going to do, Nurse Drake! I'm coming with you."

Rene looked startled, "Oh, but you *can't*, Ruby, what if you're found out? You'll have your Checks taken away and put back into Stripes to work under a junior . . . It isn't worth it, dear."

"Oh, yes it is, I'm going to risk it," I said firmly, "I just wouldn't sleep a wink anyway, thinking of you three out there on such a lovely day . . . Yes, I *will* risk it."

It was an enchanted day . . . We were in a fey mood, walking miles, talking very little. Cliff and I gathered flowers for the flat. It was very still in the heart of the woods, but a gentle breeze murmured in the tree-tops. When the sun was low it was time to leave. Cliff and Rene went on ahead; Bill and I followed leisurely. We remained silent in the harmony of understanding. The nurse-in-training was completely forgotten; I was deep in the 'hwyl'.

Suddenly Bill put his hand gently on my arm, "Look!" he whispered. I looked up and there on a branch of a tree, level with my shoulder, was a solitary robin. In lonely splendour he chirruped and chirped, the glow of the dying sun deepened the scarlet of his breast . . . A robin, a simple thing . . . a robin, the stillness, the murmuring breeze – symbols of perfection . . . Everything faded from consciousness, only the robin and ourselves remained. We felt breathlessly aware of being on the threshold of mysteries . . . Then a big bird flapped its wings overhead and startled the robin . . . He flew away and with his going the spell was broken, the magic ended. We walked on in silence both of us knowing that never would this day in Shenley Woods be forgotten.

And because of that mystic moment I missed the bus that was to get me back to my room before calling-up time!

A note on my dressing-table warned me I'd been reported to Night Sister. I flung on my uniform and raced over to the hospital where, in the dining-room I was greeted coldly by Sister:

"When you have had your breakfast, Nurse Morris, go and report yourself at Matron's office."

In spite of the coming trouble I was still in a strangely elevated state of mind; I felt nothing could harm me, nothing.

Outside Matron's office I concentrated my attention on the unknown;

I thought, if there's anything to this spirit idea, then now's the time for them to prove it. "*Don't* let her put me back into Stripes; *don't* let her make me work under a junior . . . help me, please help me." I went on muttering this under my breath until the Assistant Matron came out from her office:

"Nurse Morris, go into Matron now, please."

Inside I stood stiffly to attention, I thought, I *must* look straight into her eyes and *will* her to understand. After what seemed ages, Matron raised her eyes and looked at me – surprisingly, the iris-blue eyes were not blazing with anger:

"Your Night Sister tells me that you have not been to bed today, Nurse. Is that true?"

"Yes, Matron."

"Tell me, Nurse, why did you break such a strict rule?"

"Well, Matron, it was such a lovely day and I knew I would not be able to sleep, so I went into the country with my friends."

She was silent for a moment, regarding me closely; then with raised eyebrow she asked: "How old are you, Nurse Morris?"

"Twenty-one, Matron."

Another pause, then nodding her head slowly, she repeated:

"Twenty-one . . . Are you not *far* too dramatic for so young a girl?"

"Dramatic, Matron!" I repeated, astonished, "I don't know . . . Am I?"

Ignoring my query, she went on, "Well, Nurse, as you were on duty last night, and you've had no sleep all day, you are in no fit state to be responsible for patients tonight."

"I'm sorry, Matron."

"You will now go to Sick Bay and sleep there tonight. In the morning I will decide what's to be done about you."

"I'm sorry, Matron," I said again, and went out.

En route to the nurses' sick quarters I bumped into Husky, told her all about it and asked her to let Rene know where I was. And I popped into the nurses' sitting-room and found a tattered volume of poems.

Lying on the bed I looked in the index and found *The Ode To The Nightingale.* And as I read aloud, 'My heart aches, and a drowsy numbness pains my sense . . .' I was seized by a strange lightness which flooded my being . . . I found myself caught up and winged out into space, floating 'twixt earth and the blue dome of heaven . . . Peace and rest sublime filled my eager, released spirit. On one side the night, with crescent moon setting, three wondrous stars, brilliant on silver tip, wooed her down to rest; two close by stayed to watch the lord of day, cast to the shy clouds, colours of many hues:

Below, in the silence of the grey abyss of expectancy came the sound of fluttering wings. I watched the spiral flight of pure white doves ascending on their gentle way to heaven . . . And as the last one disappeared from sight, a sudden touch on my arm wrenched me back from that ecstatic freedom.

"Ruby, my dear," came Rene's anxious voice, "*what* happened! Was she absolutely furious?"

Feeling neither 'here' nor 'there' I opened my eyes and looked at Rene dreamily, then at my watch. I'd been on the bed less than three minutes. Then suddenly I was alert feeling as though I'd wakened from a deep, refreshing sleep . . . There was a feeling almost of bliss:

Rene shook my arm a little, "Are you all right?" she asked anxiously, "Why are you looking at me so strangely?"

How to explain such an experience? Words could not help, only confuse; so I said simply, "I've just had a wonderful experience . . . I was out of my body."

My friend's look of concern turned critically professional:

"You *must* be ill." She put her gentle hand on my forehead.

"Gracious no," said I, sitting up, "I feel absolutely wonderful, I want to go on duty."

"In that case, tell me more about it."

But at that moment in came Home Sister who shooed Rene away. She took my temperature which was normal, then tut-tutted scornfully as she confiscated my book of poems. Without a word she switched off the light, turned and closed the door behind her . . . In moments I fell into deep dreamless sleep.

For whatever reason my punishment for breaking the rule was light. I was neither put back into Stripes, nor made to work under a junior. Instead I was taken off nights and sent to Allcroft, male and female Surgical wards facing each other on the ground floor.

Sister Allcroft was a formidable character and the terror of the medical students serving as dressers on her wards. A tall, angular woman with pitch-black hair piled high atop her head, on which perched the frill cap. Her 'black-button' eyes hugged a beak of a nose set in a long, narrow face, her mouth a pale streak of sternness; heavy boots peeped from under the long dress which, being full in the back, gathered into a bustle; from a black cord around her neck hung a lorgnette. To us young nurses she seemed as old as Methuselah.

Sister Allcroft had two obsessions, firstly, to protect the young nurses in her charge from the blasting revelation of an exposed man – actually, almost all the men were very modest, but she caused them and ourselves unnecessary embarrassment, secondly, she had a passion for soft pillows which she hoarded up in the loft.

Such pillows on Allcroft proved to be as precious as Bovril, but being new on the ward I did not know this. A day came when Sister went off for her lunch, leaving the junior nurse and me to tidy beds and do 'backs'. We found a woman looking dreadfully uncomfortable and in pain, it was the second day after her major operation and she was lying awkwardly against the pillows, only two of which were soft.

Nurse Martha's keen eye saw at once the cause of the bother, she needed more soft pillows to make her comfortable. I searched in every cupboard – a host of things but no soft pillows. So I tripped up into the loft – everything there too, save pillows. Just as I turned to abandon the search my eye caught sight of a wee bit of striped material jutting out from under an ocean of blankets. I dived in and scooped out five pillows and hurried down into the ward.

When we'd finished fixing her up, she sank back against the pillows, sighed and closed her eyes. "Ah, thank you, Nurse, that feels wonderful . . . I'm sure I can sleep now."

Later, we trotted off for lunch, I mentally giving Martha a pat on the back. And returned to the ward to be greeted by a booming voice: "Nurse Morris! How *dare* you invade my loft?"

I was flabbergasted, "Invade . . . I-Invade your loft, Sister?"

"Who gave you permission to touch my pillows?"

I tried to stammer out that we'd only tried to make the patient comfortable, but with a flourish of her thin arm she bellowed:

"Go *immediately,* and put that patient back in precisely the same position as you found her . . . Return five pillows to the loft . . . GO . . ."

Trembling with rage I turned to obey.

Rene and I had quite a collection of hospital stories which we related on suitable occasions. Two such stories were about probationers. Both girls were from the heart of rural Ireland. They were completely bewildered by the routine and strangeness of the huge hospital. To a ward's Sister's constant exasperation her probationer persisted in finishing the task in hand before obeying an order. Eventually, Sister called her over to her desk and once more gave her a stern lecture about coming at once when called, either by herself, or a senior:

"Now, Nurse," she concluded, "Is it *clearly* understood? You are to come *at once* when you are called!"

"Och, yes, Sister, sure and I'm understanding, I'm to come at once."

A few days later came the test.

She had just struggled through the swing-door of Cambridge ward with the heavy can of milk which was deposited outside daily. And then came Sister's voice – loud and clear from the kitchen, "Nurse, come here . . . I want you immediately!"

The 'understanding' worked . . . Down went the pail, firmly placed on the spot, and she fled to the kitchen. At that moment, in answer to an urgent call to come to the ward, in rushed the House Physician . . . Down went the pail . . . CRASH . . . CLANG . . . CRASH . . . Down went the doctor, slithering and sliding half-way across the ward in a sea of milk.

The other nurse came to grief on a surgical ward, whose honorary surgeon was an immense figure of a man, who wore a pince-nez, which he was forever absent-mindedly taking off and putting on. Due to his height a special mat was kept in readiness for his rounds, for he often knelt at a patient's bedside in order to demonstrate some point or other to the students grouped around him.

This particular morning things were not going too well. High tension was in the ward. Little things had gone wrong, and the famous mat was not at hand. With heart all aflutter the Irish probationer kept close to Sister, straining her ears to hear any sudden command. The surgeon, while shooting questions to his flock of students, fiddled as usual with his pince-nez, and later with a pair of forceps. Presently, at the bed-side of a diminutive granny, he suddenly turned to Sister, and grunted:

"Mat, Sister."

"Mat, Nurse," hissed Sister over her shoulder.

As the nurse turned to fly for the mat the surgeon held out his hand to her and said, "Here, Nurse, boil this."

The colleen rushed away with two things in hand . . . The forceps *and* the pince-nez. The mat being foremost in her agitated mind, she tore past the sterilizer and on to the kitchen. Snatching up the mat she rushed back into the ward. The word 'boil' now came to mind, so she rushed to the sterilizer and popped the two items, clutched in her clammy hand, straight into the boiling water.

The surgeon knelt on his mat, screwed up his eyes, became aware something was missing. He turned and snapped, "Glasses, Nurse!"

The poor girl all but fainted, but blurted out:

"By all the Saints and the Blessed Virgin. Sure and 'twas yourself told me to boil them."

Thus it was that Ireland received back two of her daughters . . .

Chapter Fourteen

Several weeks later when the four of us were at the flat, we were in a serious mood, and after supper Bill chose some records and we settled down for an hour of music. As usual Martha was quickly banished by the exquisite music of Fritz Kreisler's 'Liebeslied' and 'Liebefreud'; this followed by a Beethoven concerto. I noticed Bill's hesitation before putting on the last record – Tchaikovsky's Andante Cantabile. The atmosphere immediately became more tense as the first notes flowed out into the room . . . My heart started thumping . . . Why this, why this, I thought. Don't be silly, there's nothing here.

There was an uncanny stillness when Bill took the record off and closed the cabinet lid. We remained silent as he sank back again in his chair and closed his eyes. We hoped he would recite some poems, especially 'The Ode To The Nightingale'. At that time our adoration of John Keats had almost reached the pitch of religious fervour. Sure enough he started the ode, his beautiful voice giving depth to the haunting beauty of the words. As he was saying, 'Darkling I listen, and for many a time I have been half in love with easeful Death', there came a sudden, startling interruption. At the word 'death' he gave a half-stifled gasp, up went his hand pointing to the light and from his lips came a command in a strange voice:

"Put out that light!"

We froze to our chairs not daring to move. I watched Bill's face closely; he was pale but his breathing was quiet and unhurried, but his expression unlike any I'd ever seen before: the command was repeated urgently, "Put out that light!" His eyes remained closed.

Cliff whispered to me. "Whatever can we do, Rube?"

But Rene quietly got up and switched off the light, then turned up the gas-fire. When she sat down I asked calmly, "Who are you?"

"I am Keats, the poet," said the voice.

Under such circumstances, one could hardly say, 'How do you do?' To me it was preposterous to believe that it could be the poet, but nevertheless, the idea was enchanting. One of my many failings has always been, being a 'Doubting Thomas', but in the events of the following months, it was a good thing that my training as a nurse had helped develop my latent critical faculty.

"Why have you come to *us*?" Rene asked quietly.

"These many months I have been waiting; so often have I spoken to you, but you did not hear me." But for some reason the trance ended abruptly; 'Keats' said breathlessly, "The soul of this body is returning . . . I must go . . . I will come again."

As Bill opened his eyes, Rene switched on the light. This time he was not cold nor exhausted, but seemed as though wakening from refreshing sleep. He looked at us calmly, "You don't have to tell me, I know . . . What did I say?"

There was an incredulous, wistful look in his eyes as Cliff told him: "How wonderful – if only it was true! But it can't be, I just do not believe in life after death."

But Rene, the trusting, ethereal one among us said firmly:

"Well, I believe it, I really do believe it was Keats."

I had to admit that the room was strangely tranquil, and Bill himself in a calm, elevated state of mind. But that was no proof that a spirit, either genuine or masquerading as the poet, had taken possession of him. But that evening established a routine of trances whenever opportunity presented itself. At first it only happened when we four were together, but later, it seemed inevitable that when Bill and I were alone in the flat, he would go off into a deep trance.

After a while when Cliff decided that Bill seemed none the worse after these 'visitations', Cliff lost his nervousness. The very fact that many of the personalities claimed to be a famous or renowned departed person, strengthened my theory of the subconscious demonstrating its mysterious power. But I too felt a wistful desire to believe in Keats, and at times I was nearly sure . . . But only 'nearly' and to this day I remain unconvinced. Listening to his beautiful 'talks' when he instilled into our minds the ideals of truth, beauty and love with burning sincerity, was inspiring and convincing. I asked him about life after death. He spoke of joy, peace, flowers, birds and gardens . . . In fact describing a replica of earth sans punishment, pain or grief:

"But what of hell?" I wanted to know.

"My sister," came the reply, "My sister, a good thought and a good deed goes on throughout the universe, creating more good thoughts and deeds. But evil thoughts and deeds live only until they are redeemed."

Then I asked, "Where is Bill now?"

He frowned, not seeming to understand:

"Bill . . . Bill . . .?"

"I mean, the soul of this body . . . Where is it now?"

"It has gone to my valley of nightingales."

Often I had the impression of an invisible queue waiting their turn to step into Bill's body. One evening came what seemed to me 'evidence'. We had been talking to a quite ordinary person who seemed bewildered, and begged to be taken to Joan, it was a male voice, and suddenly he'd gone and the voice and personality changed into that of a woman. She seemed grandly dramatic, the voice beautiful and she spoke in French, of which we understood only a little.

It was our routine to remain quiet as each new person came in, and then ask, "Who are you?"

This one registered great surprise, then in broken English, demanded, "You do not . . . *know*? The gr-reat Sarah Bernhardt!" She pointed at the door and tried to explain something:

"Out there, when I come – 'e flut-terrs 'is wings . . . 'ow you say – a leetle, leetle . . .? So fr-rightened when I come – 'e is in a carrge . . ." Her hands fashioned a cage.

"Oh, you mean our canary," said Cliff.

"Ca-na-ry . . ." and repeated slowly, "Ca-na-ry . . . 'ow 'arsh a name for so *beau-ti-ful* a thing . . . When I come you must covair 'im up."

We had often wondered why it was that the bird sometimes fluttered about, seemingly frightened. Now, having warned us of its fear she lost interest and reverted back to French, apparently addressing an invisible audience.

In those pre-hospital days my passion for the stage had been a tightly locked secret in my heart. Books on the subject were strictly banned from home, and so the divine Sarah was scarcely a name to me. I had no way of knowing if this personality corresponded to the real Sarah, and I don't think any of us knew if she was alive or dead.

And later on another occasion when she seemed to be acting a part, there came an amusing interruption. Suddenly while registering despair she flung up her arms and clasped her head . . . a pause, and a most puzzled expression crossed her face. Slowly, carefully, her hands felt all over the head, face, neck, then on down the body until she came to the trousered legs. She straightened, gave a most delicious little chuckle, and in English, said gaily:

"Ooh, la la! It is the body of . . . a man!"

Later, a sinister note was introduced into these sessions by a dynamic personality who claimed to be Beethoven. Some mild personality was seemingly rudely pushed out, and in came this flood of frenzy, with hands outstretched, and fingers searching frantically.

The low guttural voice stated, "I am Beethoven, Beethoven . . . Give me piano, piano, piano . . ." the while the searching fingers groped about feeling furniture, walls and sideboard. There was something frightening about the intensity of the desire to play the piano.

Rene explained we did not have a piano. And just as abruptly, with a despairing "Ach . . . so . . ." he, or it, went out.

My scepticism deepened when yet another person came and claimed to be Shakespeare. He was gentle, quietly spoken and philosophical, using 'thee', 'thou' and 'my child'.

How I regretted that we did not have a piano, for it would have been startling to say the least if Bill had suddenly played it in a Beethoven manner, especially as he did not know a note of music. During off-duty times at hospital Rene and I had long discussions about the phenomena, I ardently disputing the spirit hypothesis, while she was more than half-convinced that the flat was full of disembodied entities. I protested rather hotly, "But, Rene, why on earth should spirits of famous people bother to visit us – four very ordinary human beings? Keats, Bernhardt, Beethoven, and now even Shakespeare! It makes no sense to my mind – I just do *not* believe it. There *must* be a natural explanation."

"But, Ruby," Rene came back, reasonably enough, "if it *is* true, and millions do believe in it, why *shouldn't* they come to us? What's more natural than to seek people who love their work?"

"Could be, I suppose," I conceded grudgingly, "but what an appalling thought. Earth-bound spirits forever seeking a chance to take possession of a living person and use it to express their frustrated longings and thwarted ambitions . . . It's a repulsive idea to me . . . No, Rene, I just won't believe in it."

"Well, how about guardian angels? How do you explain them? And hauntings. And all the weird things I saw out in India, how is one to explain it?"

But I stuck stubbornly to my guns, "There *must* be a natural explanation."

However, soon after the appearance of Shakespeare, our delvings into the unknown were halted by my sudden illness and operation.

Chapter Fifteen

I should not have been surprised at the culmination of the persistent attacks of vomiting I'd suffered since coming to the hospital. Three times warded for diagnosis which brought forth an array of queries: first time – Gastritis; second time – Gall-bladder, and third – T.B. glands in the mesentery. Then came the day when, after hours of being sick in the toilet, I was found unconscious by a nurse, who raised the alarm. And the first thing I heard on regaining consciousness was Dr. Riley's voice saying:

"This has gone on long enough, Sister, medical treatment is not helping her at all . . . I rather suspect a chronic appendix . . . I'll get Mr. Cope to see her as soon as he arrives . . ." I looked up at him, "How are you feeling now, Nurse?"

"Still feeling very giddy, Sir."

Then with a stab of fear I saw Sister Eales beside me and knew then that I was in Lilian Holland, so I asked, "Why am I in Lilian, Doctor?"

"Because I want Mr. Cope to see you . . . You can't go on like this, can you, Nurse?" he answered kindly.

Mr. Zachary Cope was one of the most popular surgeons at St. Mary's, he was always kind and courteous to us nurses, and very pleasant to work with in the theatre.

When he'd finished examining me he patted my hand, "Well, Nurse, I agree with Dr. Riley that medical treatment is not helping . . . I rather suspect that appendix, I would like to do a laparotomy and have a look."

"I'm in your hands, Sir, as it is I can't get on with my training, the attacks are getting worse."

"Right – we'll do it this afternoon . . . Five o'clock, please, Sister."

It was a strange feeling lying on the trolley instead of at its side heading for the theatre. Mr. Mathews, the senior anaesthetist, smiled down at me encouragingly as he placed the mask over my face, he too was a favourite with the nurses:

"That's right, Nurse, blow it away . . . Blow it away . . ." the calm voice blended with the smothering waves of ether . . . "That's right, blow it away . . . Breathe away gently, gently . . . You're doing fine . . . fine . . . fine."

I knew no more until a burning pain in my stomach, and a vomit bowl under my chin informed me I was back in bed.

The following twenty-four hours was a blur of pain and incessant vomiting, with acute attacks of hiccoughs as a variation. Everything that was done to stop them failed, and early in the night they became so violent the night nurse hastily phoned for the house surgeon.

"Might have expected this," he grumbled, scribbling on my chart, "things always go wrong with doctors and nurses . . . Give her this at once." And off he went.

Nurse Moody gave it to me, and the almost immediate reaction startled us both. I turned deathly cold, feet and hands curled and twisted inwards, painfully – the awful feeling crept up my body and into my head, leaving tongue and neck grotesquely twisted – from head to foot I was convulsed. For a moment the nurse stared at me in horror, then she rushed to the light with the injection bottle, she nodded her head – it was the right injection. I tried to say I felt I was dying, but only broken sounds came forth.

The night nurse rushed down the ward to the phone, and in minutes an array of anxious-looking people stood at my bed-side – night surgeon, Home Sister and Matron! Suddenly, somewhere at the back of my mind the situation seemed comical; I wanted to laugh – there was I the would-be famous actress, humbly enthroned on a bedpan – all dignity fled and in the grip of convulsions. I tried to say, "Don't worry, I'm not going to die." But only a wordless jumble came out.

The attack lasted about half-an-hour, then the doctor turned to Matron, "That was a very nasty attack of tetany, Matron, but she'll be all right now, thank heaven, I'll get Mr. Cope to see her in the morning."

By the time the Surgeon arrived I'd perked up considerably, the vomiting and hiccoughs had stopped, and I was less like an overblown balloon. And I was able to take an interest in the goings-on in the ward. My bed, as a privilege to students and nurses, had red screens round it for privacy, but a small gap gave me a view down the ward. And to my delighted surprise the ward door opened and in walked my brother George, with a huge bunch of flowers. He had a word with Sister, then came to me, a large grin on his face hiding anxiety; he kissed me gently, then scrutinized me:

"Well, well, well," he said with his loving smile, "what a carryon, when Dad phoned me about Matron's telegram, I thought you were flipping-well dying . . . and here you are as bright as a button – you *are* an old fraud."

His bubbling personality asserted its usual tonic effect, I giggled weakly, "I'd no idea Matron had sent a telegram – what did she say?" I asked curiously:

"To come immediately as you were dangerously ill. Dad's in bed with flu, so I came . . . I'd have come anyway."

Sister poked her head round the screen: "Mr. Morris. Matron has phoned to say she would be glad if you could arrange to stay overnight in London."

"I've made arrangements to do that, Sister," George replied quietly.

Sister smiled warmly at both of us, "My word, you two are *so* alike – are you twins?"

"Only in spirit, Sister," said George.

I was thrilled he was staying for another day, for here was the chance for him to meet Bill and Cliff: "They're *sure* to ask you to stay the night," I told him as I gave him their address, "and I know they'll make you terribly welcome."

I waited eagerly for him coming in the morning.

He dumped his load of flowers and fruit, beaming, and I knew at once he'd enjoyed himself; "From Bill and Cliff," he said, with a twinkle in his eye, "They send their love to you and are coming to see you as soon as they can. That Bill is a scream, isn't he? My sides are still aching from laughing – he ought to be on the stage."

Then settling himself on the chair he gave me a meaningful look:

"Now, love – tell your brother George – who's in love with whom?"

As far as it was possible with a stomach full of stitches I raised myself up in bed and stated solemnly, "It's a platonic friendship."

George snorted derisively, "Oh, bosh and boloney, Rubes, a couple of good-looking chaps like that – platonic my foot!"

And I replied in earnest dignity, "It is, George, I assure you it is . . . As a matter of fact, it's on a very high level."

The twinkle deepened, and he chuckled, "Well, my dear little sister, you can't go on like that for ever, you know."

Before he left to catch his train, George said, "I *like* those two lads, Rubes, I've invited them to come for a visit to Southport, I know Muriel will love meeting them."

And in due course they went, and from that time on, my family always referred to them as the 'boys'.

I had time during the days before I went home to Prestatyn to ponder about psychic phenomena, I was so puzzled about it happening to Bill who was the most practical and level-headed of us four. His attitude to the whole thing continued to remain a mixture of resentment, irritation and fascination. But it was the fascination that kept us delving further and further. When in later years I'd told the full story to one or two people who were in Psychic Research, each asked: "Why on *earth* didn't you contact Sir William Crookes? He would have been very keen to test out such a natural medium."

The answer to that was simple – we'd never heard of such an organisation as the Psychical Research Society, nor of Sir William Crookes.

At home, during convalescence, my small sister Lilas delighted fussing over me, practising her ambition to be a nurse, 'just like Ruby'; she'd somewhere heard that feet must be propped up after an operation so whenever I sat down she staggered over with a heavy 'humpty' and carefully lifted my legs onto it.

I got back on duty in time for Christmas and was sent on night duty on Lilian Holland, and so I had to wait for my nights-off before going to the flat. It happened on that first time that Bill and I came face to face with the dangers of our experimenting and playing with fire. We were alone and Bill was soon in a trance, assuming the voice and mannerisms of 'Shakespeare'. I asked some questions and suddenly his expression altered to anxiety; he said quickly:

"This body is weary, we must not use it so often . . . It is dangerous to do this without the four elements – air, fire, earth, and water."

At which words Bill's body gave a peculiar quiver, and as I stared with alert nervousness; his expression became unspeakably evil – so evil I could neither speak nor move – I just stared. The room itself seemed full of evil. Then from Bill's lips came a flood of vicious-sounding words which I did not understand . . . Then just as suddenly the expression vanished:

"My child, my child, do not be afraid," said the gentle voice, "he has gone, he has gone."

"Gone? But who . . . *What* was it?" I whispered, "I am terribly afraid!"

His reply sounded wistful:

"Alas . . . It was my evil self." And so saying, was gone . . . Bill opened his eyes and shuddered, "Oh, I'm *so* cold . . ." And looked exactly as he had after the first trance. When I gave him some warm milk and brandy he said listlessly, "I wish we could stop these trances, Ruby, I've no resistance you know, it's all happening against my will."

"Bill, we've *got* to stop them, he told me it's dangerous to do it without the four elements of fire, earth, air and water."

"What on earth does that mean?" Bill muttered irritably.

I glanced at my watch, "Heavens, it's late, Bill, I must rush are you all right now?"

He smiled wearily, "I'm O.K. Nurse Morris . . . Don't worry, Cliff will be in soon."

But I was worried. Rene and I talked it over anxiously. We felt responsible as it was we who had started the whole thing off. And our dismay deepened when a new development came – poltergeist activities started – crockery found on the floor broken to pieces; gramophone records found in the cabinet split in half. The canary too, showed signs of panic, fluttering wildly round his cage.

Bill became more and more tired, while Cliff was plainly terrified. The whole thing was becoming beyond our control and one afternoon Cliff told me, "Rube, the flat doesn't seem to belong to us any more – it feels full of 'things'."

Warnings too from Keats, "This body is becoming weak – we will have to go."

Then, strangely, came a period when nothing happened at all, and we all relaxed, believing that whatever it was, had gone. Until one evening Bill brought home a small, pink azalea plant in full bloom; Rene teased him saying it must have cost the earth:

"I just couldn't resist it, Rene, it's so beautiful, if I'm careful it should last a few weeks." He put it on the small table by the window. Shortly after this, we four were having the usual musical evening, when most abruptly Bill was sent into trance, and there was our beloved Keats . . . He walked straight over to the azalea, paused for a long moment in silence, then stretching his hands out over it, said:

"Here is beauty – let it remain." Then came to the middle of the room with hands still outstretched, palms down; he spoke quietly:

"Here on this spot let us build a tree of beauty, truth, love and compassion."

I rather think we must have been half-hypnotised, for as he backed slowly towards the door, with arms half out beckoningly to us, Rene and I rose somewhat dazedly to follow:

He entreated earnestly, "My brother, my sisters, come with me – come to my valley of nightingales."

Cliff caught my arm urgently:

"*No*, Rube! No, Rene!"

But the sound of his voice ended the trance as abruptly as it had started: Bill opened his eyes and asked, "Why am I standing?"

We all remember vividly the next time Keats came, some weeks later.

He went straight to the spot that had been indicated for the tree to grow, gazed down at it for a moment, then said sadly:

"The tree is stunted . . . it has not grown . . . Alas, how frail is human nature!" We felt ashamed.

But it was in early spring that the evening came that for Bill and me, almost ended in complete disaster.

I had a late pass up to eleven o'clock and we were alone in the flat. Bill was happy and relaxed. We laughed a lot as we washed up the supper dishes, and Bill said with determination, "I am *not* going into a trance tonight, Ruby Morris – I'm sick of it. What's the use of our being together? I'm more absent than present!"

But later, while reading a play of Bernard Shaw's he'd only reached the bottom of the second page when the book fell to the floor; his eyes closed, his hand pointed to the light:

"My sister, put out the light."

It was the voice of Keats; I felt a stab of irritation and anger. Bill did not want to 'go off', but he had no resistance.

As soon as the room had only the light from the gas fire, the voice started warningly: "My sister, I come only to warn you." The sentence was switched off like an electric light, and to my horror Bill's body gave a spasmodical quiver as once before. It seemed as though there was an inner struggle and Keats was pushed out, his place taken by an entity of unbelievable evil, the face distorted by rage.

I have never understood the meaning of all that followed, but I will tell you exactly what happened:

Seemingly unaware of my presence he leapt up from the chair, turning his head searchingly, this way and that, then shouted in a most terrible voice: "Where is it? Where is it? Give it to me, Give it to me!"

My heart was pounding. I got up and backed cautiously towards the window. And stood watching him clawing the table, chairs, the sideboard, as hot, angry words poured forth, mostly unintelligible, in an incessant stream, with "Where is it? Give it to me", breaking in. I felt terrified for Bill's safety, and the fear caused an influx of courage – similar to that when I was guarding the patient in room seven.

And so in a hard, penetrating voice I said:

"Get – out – of – that – body, you foul thing!"

At which he swung round looking towards me with infuriated surprise: "You little bit of a thing," he hissed, "I could cr-rush you in one hand . . . Give it to me, give it to me . . ."

I ran past him towards the door, but he caught me by the throat and swung round again, his back to the wall. There we stood, he towering over me, and I struggling frantically to pull myself free. The pressure on my throat tightened relentlessly. I knew that unless help came quickly, I should be strangled:

I prayed hard; "Help me, God, please help me. Send this demon away."

My head seemed to be exploding into a red mist – when Bill's hands fell away from my throat – his body sagged and I tried to support it, at the same time taking in gulps of air. Then came a mere whisper of a voice, anguished words: "My sister, I cannot keep him out – a moment only," it was Keats, "when he comes, be brave, hold his hands and *will* it back to him . . . He . . . ahh . . ."

He was gone. The body straightened, the powerful entity was back:

"Now," he demanded, "give it to me!"

I hadn't the faintest idea what he wanted but I held out my hands and said. "Whatever it is you want, *take* it – I don't want it."

Thus we stood, the grasp on my hands like a vice, a few moments, then with a sharp intake of breath he fell heavily to the floor . . . I put on the light and looked down at him. It was the most appalling moment of my life. There he lay, rigid, motionless, and he was not breathing! Still shaking I knelt beside him. There was no pulse . . . I was stunned: "Dear God, no! Don't let him die . . . Oh, God, don't let him die!"

My first impulse was to phone for a doctor, but intuition told me to wait. And after what seemed to me a lifetime, but was probably only minutes, there came one long, slow breath . . . a pause . . . then another, and another. His pulse fluttered weakly. I cried out loud, "Thank God he's coming round, he's coming round."

His eyes opened and he stared at me without a glimmer of recognition. An expression of stark horror crept over his face, as he stared over my shoulder towards the corner by the door. Suddenly, he jumped to his feet and ran to the wall. He leaned against it and pulled himself up by the beading and gave a heart-rending cry, "Clif-ford . . . Clif-ford . . . *Clif-ford*."

I tried to pull him down, "Bill, Bill, my dear, it's all right, you're back, you're quite safe . . . Everything's all right . . . Bill!"

He looked down at me then, still without recognition. Then a frantic glance at the window, which fortunately was closed. With another loud cry he pushed me aside and ran across the room. As he struggled to open the window I tugged at his coat. I managed to pull him away and push him down into the armchair. In desperation, I slapped his face and shook him: "Will you listen to me! Pull yourself together, Bill. For heaven's sake *listen* . . . I'm Ruby . . . You're back and quite safe!"

Then he suddenly pulled himself together, looked at me, then burst into bitter sobs . . . "Oh, Ruby, it was awful, awful . . . I thought I was dead."

When we'd calmed down he told me what happened:

"I was standing over there (he pointed to the corner by the door). It seemed I'd come back from . . . I don't know, some far distance. I felt terribly lost and afraid. I called and called to you, Cliff, Rene; nobody answered. Then a terrible coldness crept through me . . . And – and I looked down at a repulsive black thing on the floor! (He pointed to the spot where he'd fallen), I stared at it and suddenly saw that it was my own body . . . I thought I must be dead," he shuddered violently, "I don't know what happened then, I only remember calling for Cliff . . ."

I went to the kitchen and poured out a large brandy. I took a hasty look at my throat, saw the red weals and bruises; I had no intention of letting Bill know what had happened, so I tied my scarf round my neck. I went back to the sitting room with the drink, and lightly remarked how long the azalea was lasting. It had not shed a single flower or leaf since Bill had bought it three months ago. Then I made tea for us. Presently, as we sat by the fire sipping it, we heard Cliff coming up the stairs. Bill said quickly:

"Not a word to Cliff about all this, he's so nervous. We'll find some way to stop it ourselves."

Chapter Sixteen

Rene's reaction when she saw the state of my throat was complete horror; she listened quietly while I related all that happened. Her eyes widened with fear and anxiety, "Oh, Ruby, love, what *have* we done?" she asked in agitation, "Surely, even *you* must believe it *is* spirits!"

I mused for a moment, "No, Rene, I still can't believe it. But who, or what 'Keats' is, and the others, perhaps we shall never know. All I do know is that I thank God for saving us."

"But what are we going to do? How *can* we stop it? What if Bill goes into trance when he's alone and that awful thing comes back? We've *got* to do something."

"We certainly have, but Rene, if we mentioned it to anyone here, they'd think us completely 'dotty'."

"Well, we're not," declared my friend stoutly, "Where could you find a better balanced or more humorous person than Bill. That's what I just can't understand – for it to be him of all people."

I suddenly felt dizzy with fatigue. I got up to go, then caught a glimpse of my throat in Rene's mirror, "Goodness, what a mess it looks, Rene, thank heaven my uniform collar will hide it; Gosh, I mustn't let Husky see it."

And on the following morning, Rene and I met at the top of the main stairway, she on her way to X-ray, and I to the dispensary.

As we hurried down the stairs, Rene said anxiously, "Do you think it would do any good if we explained to the 'people' that they are harming Bill, and beg them to go away?"

I sighed, "I somehow doubt it, but we'll try anyway."

When we reached the ground floor we noticed a very tall young man standing by the lift. His hands were in his pockets, he was gazing away into space, seemingly oblivious of everything. We glanced at him as we passed, "Never seen him before, have you?" said Rene.

"No, never."

Before we turned the corner Rene turned for another peep at him:

"Gosh, he is handsome, reminds me of a Greek god. Wonder who he is?"

"New medical student, I should think," I answered absent-mindedly.

By the time we could go to the flat again, all the marks on my throat had gone. I was in a very determined frame of mind – so was Bill. And on that occasion Bill and I came near to the only quarrel we'd ever had. Due to the attempt to put an end to his trances.

The atmosphere in the flat was almost palpable with tension.

We all sat down and Cliff fidgeted with a book. Bill was coldly calm. After a few moments of uncomfortable silence, he broke it by saying sternly, "Now, Cliff, Rene, and you Ruby, I want you to go out for an hour. I'm determined to stop going into trance. I will deal with it myself."

Cliff jumped up and caught Rene's hand:

"Come, dear," he said nervously, "I just cannot stand any more of it."

I remained seated:

"I said you, too, Ruby."

"What! Leave you alone. Don't be so absurd, Bill, of course I'm not going."

He answered slowly, stubbornly, "I am asking you to leave this flat *now*, Ruby – I'll deal with this myself."

Cliff and Rene stood waiting for me at the door:

I took a deep breath; Bill seemed determined to try and tackle something that I knew could be fatal, for how could he deal with spirits when he was not conscious. So I remained seated and said coldly, "Bill, this is your flat and you have the right to order me out of it. If you insist, I shall go. But, if I leave this flat tonight I shall *never* set foot in it again, nor shall I ever speak to you again."

And I meant it.

We stared unflinchingly at each other for a long moment, then suddenly he shrugged, and his tired face broke into a lovely smile.

"All right, Nurse Morris, you win – stay."

Cliff tugged at Rene's arm, "Oh, come on, Rene, let's go," but she held back looking unwilling and anxious.

"Rene, please do go," I urged, "Don't worry, it will be all right."

The door of the flat had scarcely closed before Bill was off.

Strangely, I felt no fear as I switched off the light – tense, but not afraid. And for a while nothing happened. Bill seemed in a deep, quiet sleep. Again I had the feeling of the invisible 'queue' of people. Then suddenly, they came – one after another.

It appeared that all, without exception, knew of our decision to stop the trances, for each and every one stated they had come to say good-bye. The trance lasted half-an-hour. The humble people said good-bye simply; the 'stars' made remarks in keeping with their personality:

"I go," said 'Sarah Bernhardt', grand, haughty and bored. "I go – to vast audience . . . I go to France, meellions 'ear my voice. That leetle ca-na-ry, 'e flut-terrs 'is wings, I don't like it . . . This body, it becomes tired . . . I go, adieu, adieu."

'Shakespeare' had more to say, ending with, "My child, farewell, and remember, I am ever near thee."

And in 'Beethoven's' voice the same urgency, the hands fluttering, the same agitation, "No piano, No piano!" Then by joining index fingers and thumbs together he made a sign in the air, making two circles, with a middle line separating them which I took to represent a capital 'B'; "If ever you need me, make this sign, call me, I shall come."

And our friend, 'Keats' was last. He too, said a lot of things that down the years proved to be true, and others not true. He was mournful and melancholy. His last words were:

"My sister, wherever you may be in the world – in sorrow, sickness, or in need. Think of me, just *think* of me. Call me, I promise you I shall come." And with a sigh, he was gone.

Bill opened his eyes; we looked at each other:

"They've gone, Ruby – I feel it!"

"Yes, Bill, they've gone. Who, or whatever they were, they've gone. I'm quite *sure* you will never go into a trance again."

Then something happened that to this day remains inexplicable. We were sitting opposite each other in the armchairs. I was thinking over all that had been said. Suddenly, a faint sound came from the side of my chair. I can only tell you that it sounded rather like tiny electric crackles. They spread in the air, seemingly rising slowly and drifting over to Bill's chair:

He whispered, "Whatever is it, Ruby?" he looked startled.

"I don't know, Bill . . . Just keep quiet, keep still."

And in minutes the whole room was filled with these tiny cracklings.

Then in less than twenty minutes it all faded away, and we were left sitting, tense and quiet. Suddenly, the flat felt EMPTY.

Over coffee later we told Rene and Cliff about it, but I kept the import of the messages to myself: "I wonder," Cliff mused quietly, "I wonder if we'll ever know what it all means. Anyway, Rube, if it is all over, then all I can say is, thank God!"

The next morning I was called to the phone in the Nurses' Home. It was Harvey, the hall-porter. "Someone wants to speak to you, Nurse Morris – seems urgent like – told him it's against the rules, but he won't take 'no' for an answer. I'll give you a couple of minutes."

It was Bill, his voice high-pitched with excitement:

"Ruby . . . you'll *never* guess. An amazing thing! The azalea! The first thing I saw this morning when I drew the curtains – the azalea. Every single bloom and leaf gone! Fallen, the plant is dead!"

And that was the end of the strange happenings at No. 5, St. Stephen's Road.

* * *

Rene and I took stock of the rest of the year with mixed feelings. We felt a wonderful sense of release from nervous tension, but at the same time filled illogically by a sense of loss and loneliness. Depressed too because Rene was due to go to the Commercial Road Maternity Hospital for her midwifery training, only a few months hence. And for me the second year and junior state exam loomed ominously on the horizon – I just had to settle down to serious study. Thus it was that one morning found me hurrying back to my ward after early lunch, all the while Martha sternly lecturing Ruby . . . 'It's no use, you know, you've just got to banish the whole thing from your mind, you'll never know why it happened, or what it all meant . . . You should be jolly thankful it's over.'

'I know, I know . . . But . . .' and at that moment I rounded a corner and collided with a heavy bump into a senior nurse:

"Sorry, Morris, old thing," she puffed apologetically.

"Sorry," I returned, "my fault. Hey, what's the matter – you look awfully agitated?"

"Should think I do! Awful morning in the theatre. Poor old Zachary – everything went wrong!"

"What happened?" said I with sympathy, knowing those frightful days in theatre when things go wrong.

"Emergency appendix . . . nearly died on the table!"

"Heavens, how ghastly! What happened?"

"Oh, the patient stopped breathing . . . terrible flap . . . had to do artificial respiration; touch and go for a while – medical student too of all things!"

"Oh, my goodness – is he all right, now?"

"Thank heaven, yes, they've just warded him in Zunz."

"Who is he?"

"Mr. Dymond."

"Dymond? Never heard of him."

The theatre nurse pursed her lips, "Never heard of Dymond! My dear, he's the cat's whiskers at rugger and boxing!" she said it as though that explained everything.

"Oh, well," I laughed, "I don't know a thing about games, I suppose that's why." We hurried away from each other.

The following morning Sister made only one announcement after breakfast, "Nurse Caffery was taken ill during the night; Nurse Morris will replace her in Zunz."

Zunz was a male and female surgical ward at each end of a short corridor. I felt a qualm of nervousness suddenly being promoted to acting staff nurse, especially knowing about the new patient – medical student, Mr. Dymond. The two junior nurses on the ward were, Nurse O'Halleron, whose thick Irish brogue was complicated by a lisp, and a dark, attractive girl from the West Indies whose name I have forgotten.

On entering the men's ward I went over to say 'good-morning' to Mr. Dymond, and was confronted by a pair of blue-grey eyes which I felt sure I'd seen before. Yes, of course, the patient was the tall young man Rene and I had seen by the lift with the faraway expression. It was a face remarkable in its contrasts in repose, sombre, almost brooding;

transformed by a lovely smile which was warm, sympathetic and friendly – altogether a charming smile.

He greeted me with a cheerful 'good-morning', his voice too was friendly and warm. Our only conversation during the first three days was 'Good-morning', 'Good-night' and, 'Are you quite comfortable?'. He was an excellent patient, quiet and considerate, and his recovery was uncomplicated; he was none the worse for his close brush with death.

It was Nurse O'Halleron who first broke the ice of professional reserve. On a morning when we were making his bed she suddenly remarked:

"Och, and I'm tired of callin' you Mr. Dymond – and what would your mother be callin' you?"

He grinned and suddenly looked very young, unprotected:

"Guess I must have been an unwanted child – it's Elmslie Chalmers."

"Och and away with you," said the Irish nurse, "I can't be fashed callin' you that –'tis death to me tongue, sure and it is – I'll call you Jimmy."

And so, unofficially, Jimmy he became.

When Nurse O'Halleron found out that he was of Irish extraction she was delighted, and I was shaken from my inborn reserve when he laughingly added:

"Actually, I'm Chinese-Irish – I was born in China."

"China!" I echoed, "Oh, h-how interesting."

"I suppose so, Nurse, but I'm afraid I don't remember much about it. I came home when I was eight."

When Mr. Cope did his round, he looked at his student patient, then at me, and said smiling, "This little nurse too gave us a nasty fright, but *she* had the decency to wait until she was back in the ward!" Then he asked kindly, "Are you feeling quite strong now, Nurse?"

I went hot with embarrassment, but felt thrilled he'd recognised me, "Yes, thank you, Sir, I feel fine."

Later, as we were tidying beds our special patient remarked:

"*That's* a coincidence, isn't it? Both branded by the same surgeon's knife."

And when he was allowed out of bed it was soon apparent that he was a very high-spirited, flirtatious young man. Hearts were all aflutter over the tall, handsome figure. The most smitten was the Irish night nurse, who was soon confiding in me her ardent hopes, and before long I was acting as liaison for the furtherance of the romance. Meanwhile I had much ado maintaining discipline in the ward; oftentimes catching him flirting with the West Indian nurse when he was supposed to be resting.

A day came when I considered things were getting a little out of hand. I came into the ward just as he was chasing the same nurse and squirting water at her from a hypodermic syringe; I curtly ordered him back to bed; but patience was stretched to the limit when I found him teaching her the Charleston. This time I addressed him acidly:

"*Mr.* Dymond, would you be *so* kind as to get *back* into bed, and *stay there*! I do not wish to report you to Sister. Please do not force me to!" And so saying I swept out of the ward.

However, in spite of the haughty Nurse Martha, as the days went by I gleaned the outline of Elmslie Chalmers' parents, which seeped into my mind, and where at night sometimes too tired to sleep, my romantic imagination conjured up fascinating pictures.

It was in 1887 that young Frank Dymond and Samuel Pollard – about whom, in later years, books were to be written – felt an urgent call to go out to China as missionaries. In due course the Bible Christian Church bade these ardent young Protestants farewell, and wished them good luck, knowing they would need it as they were being sent to Chaotung, in Yunnan in South-West China. As yet a new field barely touched by missionary work. At that time it was considered expedient for foreign missionaries to adopt Chinese dress and to grow a queue. And so until they could grow their own, the young men called upon the ingenuity of a hairdresser to make them a false queue, and this was firmly attached to the inside of a tightly fitting skull cap, which, when indoors was hung on a nail in the wall like a hat. They were housed in an insecure house with wooden fronts and white-washed mud walls, in a back street of Chaotung city, a thousand miles from the China coast, and ten thousand miles from home. In 1888 Chaotung was, of all the other cities in the area, the least attractive. Outside the city walls brigandage was rife in the mountains. Anti-foreign feeling always lurked in the atmosphere, and in particular missionaries were feared and hated, and the Chinese let them know in no uncertain terms that they wished they'd go back home.

But undaunted, these courageous men carried on trying to spread the gospel. Later, the hazards and hardships of their lives was lightened when they married. Frank Dymond's bride was a radiantly beautiful girl from New Zealand, Maud Cannon, and she shared the same ambition to carry the gospel to the diverse Chinese tribes scattered in the hills. Seven children were born of the marriage, Elmslie being the fourth son; the children wore Chinese dress, spoke Mandarin and pidgin English. Then the problem of education finally arose and there was the inevitable family upheaval. It was Maud who had to face the weary, hazardous trek through the mountains and down to the Yangtze River, and on to Shanghai by house-boat and junk, there to embark on a homeward bound ship to England, the journey in those days took six months.

I built up vivid pictures in my mind's eye, seeing the small gallant woman confronted daily with dangers from hostile tribes, brigands, and diseases such as small-pox, cholera, plague and leprosy. Elmslie Dymond was eight years old when he and his two sisters started on the long journey with their mother. Food supplies were renewed at crowded market-places – rice, fish, fruit and vegetables. The picturesque cities were set among the high mountains. The immense, natural beauty was enhanced by Buddhist temples perched on craggy, precarious prominences, and stately white pagodas dotted about whose purpose was to placate the spirits of turbulent wind and water. The progress of the journey depended on the rise and fall of the rapid river which every year took its quota of human lives. A Chinese poet wrote, "The passage to heaven is easier than that of the Yangtze Gorges."

The Dymond children had inevitably absorbed much of the Chinese way of thinking and living, so it was not difficult to picture their bewilderment and confusion on entering the confines of a boarding school. They were regarded as foreigners by their fellow pupils who delighted in yelling after them:

"Chin, chin, Chinaman, muchee muchee sad; mees aflaid all de tlade's velly, velly bad . . ."

The ditty made the Dymond boys' blood boil, the Irish blood was stirred, many fights and bloody noses were the result. As I lay in bed thinking on all these things and seeing the magnificent ranges of wild-looking mountains, covered with rhododendrons; watching the colourful Buddhist temples and yellow-robed monks, the beauty faded, to be replaced by visualising the horrors, the foul smells, insanitary conditions and loathsome diseases; I muttered turning over restlessly, "No, *indeed,* you'd never catch *me* in a place like that.

And then one day when I was in one of my 'black pit' moods with Ruby arguing fiercely with Martha on the problems of pain, cruelty and the suffering of children, I confided some of these thoughts to the sympathetic Mr. Dymond. But we were interrupted before I had time to warm to my subject; as I turned to leave the ward he said gently:

"You seem very depressed tonight, Nurse, there's never time to talk about these things, why not tell me all about it on paper?"

Which, after pondering about it, I did.

His reply revealed some aspects of his character:

Here was a person, who like myself hid behind several faces. In the eyes of the hospital Elmslie Chalmers Dymond was considered a 'tough guy', pleasure-loving, reckless and a great athlete, one who laughed in the face of trouble and pain. No-one, just no-one would be allowed to know of the misery that was within him; I turned back two pages and re-read: 'It is evident that we are both oppressed in the same way; I mean this, that inanimate things help rather than oppress us. We seem to be surrounded by people who are absolutely soulless, and although this realisation once caused me pain, I am now beginning to think it should make me immensely happy. If an appreciation of nature, music, friendship, dreams, and in fact everything that raises our life above the par of a mere animal existence, is going to make me wretched, then there must be something wrong, either with my ideals or my application of them.

'Don't you think that you and I just lack one thing? That quality one is always afraid of leading towards smug complacency – I mean contentedness. How I hate the word; it conjures up images of unfulfilled dreams and thwarted ambitions, a clouded eye and a smug suburban villa. And yet it is a thing we *must* cultivate. I am dreadfully conscious of perhaps writing platitudes, but you surely realise that your work, with all its tirednesses, and heart-breaking experiences, is one of the finest in the world.'

And the letter ended, '. . . I believe in God and *now* know him to be a God of justice as well as love. It is my fervent hope that He gives you all the beauty in life that you deserve, Jimmy.'

Before being discharged from the ward he asked me shyly:

"May I call you Ruby, and *please*, will you come out with me for coffee one morning?"

This was a startling request for in the Twenties no nurse in training was allowed to talk to students, let alone go out with one, and to do so was running the risk of instant dismissal from the hospital. So I hesitated before replying; "I'd love to," I started feeling equally shy, "b-but, how can we manage it? We daren't be seen together!"

"That's easy, I know a nice cafe in Kensington called the Blue Cat, I've never seen anyone there from Mary's; so why not let's meet there?"

This new friendship set me all aglow with ambition to pass my exams at a higher grade, and when the second year exams came along, I sat them in the usual state of nervous dithers, and achieved two ‘B’s. Over which there was much rejoicing at the flat. Clifford had recovered his natural gaiety, but after supper he suddenly fell silent, then said with a quick sigh: “Isn’t it wonderful not having any more worry over Bill”, then a quick change, “By the way, Rube, why don’t you bring your young man over to see us?”

I was instantly on the defensive, “He’s *not* my young man, it’s a platonic friendship, same as ours.”

Bill gave me a searching look, “Is it?”

“*Of course*,” I said, perhaps too heartily.

“Methinks the lady doth protest too much,” quoted Cliff teasingly.

“Anyway, Ruby, dear,” his friend cut in, “bring him along. We want to meet him.”

By this time Jimmy and I had managed a few morning coffees at the Blue Cat, during which times I had brought forth my high-flown ideas on the nice cool pinnacles of platonic friendship; giving as an example, a glowing account of Rene’s and my friendship with Bill and Cliff. To which he listened with an enigmatic expression, and when one day I’d ended somewhat breathlessly, he remarked quietly:

“So . . . You want us to be platonic friends?”

“Oh, yes, please.”

“O.K.” he said shortly and changed the subject.

In those early days of friendship with the idealistic student, I felt no inclination to tell him about the psychic ‘happenings’. I felt that his medical studies would force him to ‘pooh-pooh’ the whole thing, passing it all off as hysteria, hallucinations and wishful thinking, or interpret it in terms of psychological jargon. So instead, I coaxed him to talk more about his life; he, like Rene, had been reared in the ‘life is real, life is earnest’ school of thought, and whilst laughter in itself was not wicked, frivolity was to be regarded with suspicion. In comparison to the strict rules of conduct meted out constantly to my two medical friends, my own childhood had been free and easy.

All the things at which my friend, Jimmy, excelled – drawing, painting, sports and in particular boxing, these were regarded by his family as unworthy of serious consideration. And so he was forever torn between conflicting emotions. His love of nature gave him a longing to be a forester, but the greater pull was to dedicate his life to art. And when one day he rather shame-facedly confessed he had never wanted to be a doctor, I was dumbfounded:

"You too! *I* never wanted to go in for nursing!"

He murmured, "Same surgeon's knife. Same 'round pegs in square holes'. . . hmmmmm!"

"But why are *you* doing it?"

"I don't know really," he started slowly, "my brother Frank's influence perhaps – and family persuasion. Frank's crazy about medicine, thinks nothing else worthwhile. Wonderful chap, magnificent athlete. Beats me into a cocked hat! As soon as he's qualified he's going back to China – my sister too, in fact the whole family is nuts on China."

"And you?"

"Haven't a clue . . ."

I went on probing, "How did you go on during the war?"

"The war? Well, one thing made me piping mad, I was too young to join up – my three brothers did of course. Mother got home just before it started; she set up home for us. How she managed to cope with seven enormous appetites I cannot imagine; she was wonderful. Then when my eldest brother, John, was killed it just about broke her up. He was the apple of her eye. Then I couldn't stick it any more and ran away from home to join up; but Frank found out in time and yanked me out of the recruiting office and promptly gave me a good licking for worrying mother. How did you go on?"

I felt my face burning, "I'm ashamed to confess it, but most of it passed over my head; I was still reading fairy-tales, and they were more real to me, so it didn't make much impression on me. But my most vivid memory was in Rhyl where we were living at the time – I became the troops' mascot."

"How come?"

"Well, Rhyl was flooded by the boys and I used to take our sheep dog, Rossie, and go onto the promenade and drill with the soldiers, always standing apart from them. When they marched smartly up and down, so did Rossie and I, and at the command of 'Halt', Rossie would promptly sit down on her bobtail. And it all ended by us being made their mascot. Dad was presented with a photo of us placed in the centre of a large group of soldiers, with the inscription 'To our little Welsh mascot and her dog, Rossie'. That was my war."

"And after Rhyl?"

"Oh, we were forever moving about – Birmingham, Blackpool, Prestatyn, which is now still my home. My brother George went over to France, but came back safely – we were very lucky, only lost one cousin."

And so, over innumerable cups of coffee at 'The Blue Cat', we came to know a lot about each other's lives. And it became embarrassingly obvious to me that I had once more made a friend who was brilliant at theory. It filled me with awe seeing the ease at which this young man sailed through exams with top honours. A man capable of intense concentration, but one. who, on the impulse of the moment was capable of disappearing to the other end of the earth.

His rebellion against a medical career started at eighteen when he fled from his university at Bristol and joined a group of men emigrating to Canada on a farming scheme. The steerage fare was three pounds, and with empty pockets and high hope, off he sailed.

During the following two years his adventures would fill a book, even my over-active imagination found it difficult to keep pace with the endless variety of jobs he took to keep from starving. Those were the days of the American hobo who 'rode the rods' from one end of the continent to the other. After finishing his time on the Canadian farm, he joined the ranks of the hobos and 'bummed' from Halifax to San Francisco, dropping off here and there to pick up a job. The cups of coffee became a mirror wherein I saw exciting scenes . . . A tall, lanky man leaping onto the fast-moving freight train and hanging on to the rods for dear life . . . The 'jump-off' when the train slowed to a halt at the water-tanks; and the scramble back through clouds of steam when it got under way again. I saw the tense, furtive figure hiding under the train, in a caboose; felt the sweating fear of the 'bulls', whose job it was to find hidden adventurers, and who often delighted in shooting such a find, like a bird on a bough.

He learned to run fast, think and act in a flash, and to live with fear, working in lumber camps, tree-topping; on farms, stoking and threshing; worked with a rock, sand and gravel plant. In Eugene, Oregon, he helped lay pavements near the university and there surreptitiously set down his initials in the wet concrete. There were striking examples of disinterested kindness from total strangers. One such time was on arrival at Eugene, he stood outside a cafe, trying to ignore the awful pangs of hunger, with only a nickel in his pocket.

Presently, a young man strolled over to him and asked casually: "Care for the makings?"

"Thanks, I could certainly use it." He took the proffered paper and tobacco.

"Down on your uppers, Limey?"

"Yes," admitted 'Limey' shortly.

"Then I guess you could use these . . ." he handed over a week's supply of food tickets. "Meet you here tomorrow in the morning. I can get you a job, that's for sure . . . So long . . ."

Olsin Murray of Eugene, Oregon, was as good as his word, and furthermore, his family invited the 'limey' to come and room with them; he stayed with them for six months and formed a life-long friendship.

Another memorable event was when an old, grizzled darky, who was testing the brake-boxes and couplings, found a 'quarry' frozen to the rods. His job wasn't worth a dime if he failed to hand over to the 'bull' any hobo, and on this terrible winter's night there was one whose hands and feet would not unlock when the moment came to jump off at the water tank. The Negro and white man regarded each other for a long moment, then 'Limey' smiled: "Guess I've had it!"

But the darky took a cautious look round, then gave a wide toothsome grin: "Quiet, sah, keep quiet!" Gently he loosened the stiff limbs and carried the half-frozen man into a shed, and with experienced fingers massaged the limbs into circulation. Then brought him scalding coffee, and later bundled him into a truck and hid him under a heap of old sacks. As he quietly jumped down from the truck, this good Samaritan whispered, "Good luck, sah."

Jimmy Dymond loved the Murray family, and Oregon. They did their best to persuade him to stay on there, and he was inclined to do so. But letters from home gnawed at his conscience. They urged him, and pleaded with him to come home and continue with medicine. A final appeal from his mother turned the scale. He rode the rods down to San Francisco, and hung about the docks until he finally got a job as assistant cook on the S.S. *Lockatrin.*

Eventually, back at university he settled down and worked as though not a moment had been lost. In due course he sat for his second year exams, and passed them all without difficulty. Thrilled at this success the family decided they would like him to finish his training at St. Mary's Hospital.

Chapter Seventeen

And now here we were, the two of us, Jimmy struggling along with the problem of getting through to his finals on slender finances that meant sixpenny dinners, missed meals and tightening of the belt; while I pressed on imbibing knowledge that either bored or shocked me. But it was not long before my friend, Jim Dymond, became something of a will-o'-the-wisp in my life. By now he was a welcome visitor to the flat, for both Bill and Cliff had warmly welcomed him into the fold. And on one mellow morning there, with just the two of us, I took courage to tell him a little of the less frightening 'happenings', at which his eyes widened with stark horror, he almost gasped:

"Ruby," he started in dead earnest, "Ruby, you should just hear my mother on these subjects – trances and the like – after all her experiences in China nothing will shake her conviction that they are the works of the devil. You've been playing with fire!"

Privately thinking that the devil hypothesis an unlikely theory to explain all psychic phenomena, thereafter I left the subject alone; but surely I ruminated it was not the devil that had rescued me from that frightful predicament and saved Bill and myself from complete disaster. But what the force was that did intervene is still a mystery to me to this day.

The first will-o'-the-wisp departure came about four months later, when suddenly one morning Jim announced that his mother, having returned home from China to be with her family wanted him to return to his university in Bristol. I found myself more upset by his imminent departure than I cared to admit, even to myself. We spent our last evening together at the Piccadilly Corner House, and there to the strains of 'No, No, Nanette'; 'The Desert Song'; and heart-rending selections, such as Tosti's 'Goodbye' and others guaranteed to stir the emotions, quite suddenly I found myself unable to swallow the sumptuous meal of baked beans on toast.

It seemed that Jim too was having a similar difficulty for he was fidgeting about restlessly. I wondered vaguely if he had indigestion and just as I was about to ask him if he felt all right, he started speaking in a strangled kind of whisper: "Ruby, I've done what you asked me . . . P-played this platonic friendship game for what it's worth . . . B-but now . . . Now I want you to know that as far as I'm concerned it is no longer platonic . . . W-would you consider becoming engaged to me?"

I was rendered speechless and sat staring down at that horrible plate of beans which unaccountably seemed to be weaving about and my heart thumped sickeningly. It seemed an age before I could force myself to look up at him, and looking straight into those pleading blue-grey eyes a strange thing happened – I saw myself standing beneath the dome of a huge, austere cathedral – alone. The vision faded abruptly; I stammered, "I-I . . .", but he cut in urgently:

"Please, don't say anything now. Think about it. My train leaves Paddington at ten-thirty; it's your morning off, isn't it?

I nodded dumbly:

"Good, then let's meet at the Lyon's for coffee . . . nine-thirty, O.K.?"

Not another word was said about friendship and love. I got back to the nurses' home in a daze of fatigue and spent the night tossing and turning, thoughts whirling dizzily through my mind . . . Engaged! I become engaged to a medical student hoping to qualify as a doctor! Oh, no, no, impossible, I was going out to India with Rene . . . On and on throughout the night. And in the morning at the appointed time I tottered down Praed Street, feeling exhausted. I half expected my would-be fiancé to be looking full of divine rapture . . . But no, not so at all! He looked as cool as the proverbial cucumber.

Over the coffee cups we spoke spasmodically about nothing in particular; after the third cup I began to wonder if I'd suffered hallucinations the night before. Finally, Jim glanced at his watch; "Lummy, I must dash or I'll miss my train." Then outside, standing at the kerb edge he looked down at me tensely and in clipped tones asked: "Well, Ruby, what is the answer?"

I blinked back hot tears, then heard myself whispering tremulously:

"I-I th-think I should like to become engaged to you!"

The thin, strained face broke into a lovely, boyish smile; he grasped my hands and chuckled gleefully; "Well now, what d'you know! Ain't life *wonderful,* ain't life *simply great*? I'll write to you . . . Bye!" And so saying he dashed across the road and disappeared into the Underground.

I walked bemusedly back to hospital and up to my room where I met Rene. I stared at her and as from some far distance, said: "Hello, Rene . . . I . . . I think I'm engaged to Jimmy!" To which the ever romantic Rene responded with:

"Oh! Ruby, love, how simply lovely!"

Thus it was that letters flowed back and forth between London and Bristol. It seemed to me that Jim and I came to know more about each other through the medium of letters than if we'd been together. Eyes are said to be the mirrors of the soul, so also can letters be. Our lengthy epistles revealed similarities and diversities in our temperament. Fundamentally we were similar in that we were both emotional and imaginative; outwardly undemonstrative, inwardly religious, with the difference that I was born with a completely unorthodox mind, forever asking awkward questions. Both of us were fiercely independent, and apt to rebel against authority.

We had entered hospital life without the protection of worldly knowledge and painfully thrust into the intolerance and cruelty of life. Sickness and suffering assumed too great a proportion; the sudden contact with pain and evil robbed us of our youth, turning us into 'young-old' people. Those letters were pathetically naïve and soul-searching. Jim's were eloquent and idealistic to an extreme, but at the same time revealed a young man not yet come to terms with himself. In the 'twenties men were less sophisticated than are the present generation, too much show of emotion was considered bad form, and there was very little freedom. Subjects which are today discussed with such shattering frankness were strictly taboo. And so our journey into love was rather a case of the blind leading the blind. The thoughts we exchanged were beyond the scope of our experience, and so through pain and suffering we laid the foundation for abiding affection.

Love through the medium of letters was all very well, but on the day a letter came informing me that the Dymond family were coming to live in London I was flung into a state of panic. I re-read the alarming paragraph: ". . . My brother Frank has now passed his finals and is to do his tropical diseases at the London School. It's been arranged for me to carry on at St. Mary's . . . oh, I'm *so* excited . . . You will love mother, she's such a darling. I call her my little lady of the chimney corner; I don't know which of the two of you is the smaller!" The rest of the letter gave me the feeling that he was just as nervous as I at the thought of our meeting.

Week after week swept by with my moods fluctuating up and down, at times happy, thrilled and excited; at others full of gloom and depression. At long last there I was on my way to Kensington Gardens to meet my fiancé, all aflutter not knowing how I would feel. But I needn't have worried for all negative emotions fled at the sight of the tall, athletic figure, now filled out and even more handsome, beaming his famous smile. But he looked cool and friendly:

"Hello, Ruby," he remarked casually.

"Hello, Jimmy," said I gazing away into the distance.

However, shyness soon flowed out and happiness in as I listened to the spate of family news. I was glad not to have to talk.

Instead I watched the mind's inner picture of the Dymond family building up into a glowing story of success – it seemed to me that their house must be swaying with its load of medals, awards, cups and shields, for the Rev. Dymond's children seemed to excel at academic study and all games. I heard too about the time when Tex O'Rourke came over to Britain from America seeking a new 'white hope', and to the utter consternation of the minister and his wife, Maud, he chose their son Elmslie. All coaxing failed to budge the parents who sternly forbade Mr. O'Rourke to encourage the eager young man to return with him to America.

By this time I had become adept at watching, listening and learning; the habit of 'people-watching' persists to this day. But at that time I had but few gifts to bring to our relationship – a half-trained voice, no experience other than peculiar psychic ones and a capacity for friendship. In due course the dreaded moment came when I was invited to tea to 'meet the family'. Jim escorted me over to their house at Clapham Common, and I felt in a strait-jacket of shyness and reserve. It turned out to be an afternoon of intense interest to me. I managed to get through the lovely tea spread on an exquisite hand-embroidered Chinese tea-cloth without spilling my tea, or otherwise disgracing myself. And afterwards sitting before the glowing fire, Frank, obviously in an attempt to make me feel at home, brought out the family albums of photographs.

Faraway places; faraway people! How they had fascinated me for as long as I could remember. I relaxed as I became lost in the array of page after page of photos – scenes of China – great mountainous ranges in Yunnan Fu; photos of the humble chapel in Chaotung, and others in the country around Chaotung. There were pictures of the mighty Yangtze river, others of curling rivers; lakes, temples and pagodas. The dress of the hill tribes was quaint, in particular the Miao, among whom the Rev. Frank and Maud Dymond had done such outstanding work. All wore full petticoats below the knee, with striped woollen stockings and black cloth slippers; wide-sleeved shawl with intricate patterns draped over the shoulder. Between married and unmarried women the hair styles differed, the former wearing a high cone draped in cloth at the base, this was supposed to stay that way until death. The maidens had several flat coils atop their heads with long straight side-pieces, and through the pierced lobes of the ears hung long leather ear-rings in wide loops. They all carried men's large black umbrellas upside-down. Their round chubby faces wreathed in smiles were enchanting.

The Dymond family photos intrigued me for to me it seemed they all looked Chinese, especially the children, where most of them at toddler age wore Chinese clothes. There was one that I would love to have had for my own – father all complete with long silk gown, skull-cap and long pigtail over one shoulder; mother too in lovely silk embroidered gown and embroidered soft-soled slippers. Then turning a page, there was a most beautiful face, almost startling beauty – this was Maud Cannon taken in New Zealand as a young belle of society. The Dymond children always spoke of how mother had been engaged seven times before the sudden decision to go out to China as a missionary! This dramatic announcement to her wealthy family so enraged them she was never forgiven, she rode the storm with unshakeable determination and out she went to China, and very soon met the young man with the burning zeal, fell deeply in love with him and married him. Books have been written of those courageous missionaries, a number of whom were murdered during the Boxer rebellion. Beside the picture of the young Maud, was the young Frank Dymond, his sensitive face was that of the born idealist, highly aesthetic with steadfast eyes. His son, Frank, was very like his father . . .

All too soon it was time for me to go back to hospital. I thanked my hostess feeling rather in a dream; I was overawed by the small dignified lady whose face still held much of the beauty of her youth, the little gallant woman who had survived so many adventures in China.

With that hurdle over, having met the 'Chinese' Dymonds, the time had come for Jim to meet the Welsh Morris's. His visit to my home in Prestatyn was arranged for the last week of my holiday. I was feeling a little nervous about his reception because Father's letter, in reply to mine telling him my unofficial fiancé had been born in China, was very cautiously phrased. And from my sister Cassie I received an amusing letter in which she said the rumour had spread like wildfire through Father's home village of Llanuwchllyn that George Morris's daughter was going to marry a Chinaman. According to Cassie it went something like this:

"Good morning to you, Evans bach," remarked old Bob the boot as he met his friend at the village pump, "a fine morning it is, indeed," a quick turn of his rheumy eyes, "Have you *heard* the news!"

Evans bach yawned; "A fine day it is, Bob . . . No, nothing special like I've heard."

"Nothing special! George Morris's daughter!"

"George's daughter?" ears all alert, "Deuch, which one, Bob – what's up?"

A dramatic pause, "*Ruby* . . . She's going to marry a CHINAMAN."

Dai Evans gasped, "A Ch-Chinaman! It's not true, don't believe a word of it!"

"True it is, bach, true it is . . . Jane Jones *knows* . . . She was *told*."

"Diar Annwyl!"

"I always said," went on old Bob, scratching his tousled head, "always did say that daughter of George's was a rum one – remember the day when Kate Edwards had the South Wales minister to tea? The whole village saw her *actually pumping the pump on a Sunday*! I always said she'd come to no good, around twelve she was – old enough to know better, isn't it? A Chinaman . . . Well, well . . . Diar Annwyl . . . A CHINAMAN . . . Twt, twt . . ."

And that year Wales to me seemed more magical than ever.

But on the day that Jimmy was due to arrive the omens were not auspicious. It was gloomy and pouring with rain. I felt gloomy too; what if my family did not like him; worse still, what if he did not like them or Wales. The day dragged on until it was time for me to go to the station to meet his train. It was still raining and the train was half-an-hour late, and then when it finally steamed in . . . Lo, he was not on it! Straightaway I was flung into panic, and saw sudden death or some crippling disaster. I rushed home, for surely there would be a telegram; but no, nothing. Around eleven and with leaden feet I was going up the stairs to bed, when a knock came at the front door . . . ah . . . a telegram! I flew down the stairs, opened the door and . . . there was Elmslie Dymond, all sweetness and smiles, looking very smart in plus-fours and fawn golf-stockings.

It was those stockings that was the cause of the bother. He was greatly agitated at the discovery that the only pair of stockings that would match the plus-fours were full of holes. But Curly, the hall porter had saved the day by suddenly appearing out of the blue with a pair of stockings to give to his hero, Mr. Dymond, whom he considered a fine, upstanding young man, and worshipped him as a champion amateur boxer. Curly had paid sixpence for the stockings at an open-air market: "Might come in 'andy for your holiday in Wales, sir," he explained. A godsend but the snag was they were shop worn and grubby, hence the hasty washing and desperate hand-drying in front of the gas-fire – and thus the missed train.

Father was very impressed with his future son-in-law's charm and gaiety. Being a hypochondriac – of the more cheerful variety – Father had a wonderful time discussing his various aches and pains; his pockets always held a generous supply of pills – little pills, big pills, white and coloured – he was not to be caught out in any emergency! Twice I went into the lounge in time to hear him saying: "Don't know what it is, Jim. but I don't *quite* feel myself today – you know, niggling pain in my back, dull headache . . . D'you think I'm sickening for something? I've tried these . . . and these . . . What's your opinion? Think they're any good?"

And with a grave, professional air the medical student took the various bottles of pills and studied the labels with serious intent. Then gave forth his opinion as to the merits or demerits of the drugs of whose names he'd never heard. Oh, yes, my father heartily approved of Elmslie Dymond. And Jim responded whole-heartedly to the warmth and friendliness of my family; he loved them *and* Wales, and so passed muster. My young sister Lilas fell in love with the six foot two stranger from London. Mutual admiration was in the air – all was well in Prestatyn.

And then Father decided it was time to dispel the rumours in Llanuwchllyn. He drove us to Cassie's home at Plas Deon. Soon after our arrival there and Father and Gret had gone up to 'Hendre Mawr' to see Nain, a note came over from Mrs. X Chapel House inviting us over to tea. As Cassie re-read the note I noticed a mischievous twinkle creep into her eyes. She turned to Jimmy and asked:

"Are you a sport, Jim?"

He grinned but answered cautiously, "Well, I hope so . . . But why do you ask?"

"Just a minute," said Cassie brightly, then she tripped away up the three flights of stairs to the attic, and presently returned with a black beret and a long black pigtail under her arm: "It's Myfanwy's," she explained, "it'll do fine . . ." Then she rummaged in a drawer and brought out her box of theatrical make-up. Cassie was an artist at make-up:

The penny dropped:

"Crikey!" exclaimed Jim in alarm, "You're surely not expecting me to go out to tea dressed up as a Chinaman!"

"Just that," said Cassie smoothly, while her two children, Dorothy and Harold danced up and down with glee, "they believe you are Chinese, can't see why we can't play a joke on them – give them something to talk about . . . Now keep still."

By the time she'd finished with him he looked alarmingly Chinese, the queue was firmly attached inside the beret, his eyes and brows had an artful slant, the final touch was the long-sleeved jacket. Jim hunched up his shoulders, tucked his arms in the sleeves, bowed low to us and squeaked: "Can do, Missy?"

When we had controlled our hysterics we all trooped solemnly down the long drive and on to Chapel House which was next door. A rosy-cheeked maid opened the door, and at one look at the 'Chinaman' she fled to the back of the house. We stepped inside the hall, then along came our hostess, Mrs. Chapel House, with calm, dignified tread; Cassie introduced Jimmy and he shuffled forward, bowed low and murmured a few Mandarin phrases. The poor lady turned puce in the face, but bravely said: "How do you do . . . Please do come along to the parlour."

There was a nice, cheerful fire glowing, and the tea-table was laden with cakes, thin bread and butter, light-cakes and scones and strawberry jam. Jim sat on the edge of his chair while Cassie chatted away merrily as though all was perfectly normal. But it soon became too much even for her, she burst out laughing. Jimmy relaxed and rose from his chair and went over to our hostess and said with his most winning smile: "I'm *so* sorry, it was just a silly joke . . . Do please forgive us, I'm no Chinaman, my name's Jim Dymond."

But the lady was not amused – she never forgave us.

Later we went up to the farm as Nain insisted she must see Ruby's young man. She was in bed rosy-cheeked and smiling. Her wise old eyes crinkled up in instant approval.

Before we went back to London I had a word with Gret who had not yet voiced her opinion; "Well, Gret," I asked her a little anxiously as she was picking roses in the garden, "*You* haven't said anything! What do you think of him?"

"Well, Ruby bach, if you really want my opinion," she too had wise eyes, "if you really want it, here it is. Your life with Jimmy Dymond won't always be smooth, but it will never be dull; I'd rather starve with that one than live in comfort with many . . . I think he will be my favourite son-in-law."

Chapter Eighteen

Rene was packing to go down to the East End when I dashed into her room on my return to hospital. Husky and I felt depressed by the breaking-up of what our fellow nurses called 'The Three Musketeers'. And after her departure another will-o'-the-wisp episode swept into my life with shattering suddenness. The Dymond family had returned to China and shortly after, Jim had discovered that there was not enough money in the bank to enable him to carry on with medicine. This alarming situation he had kept to himself until other drastic arrangements had been made. I had not sensed that anything was wrong for his characteristic sunny smile almost always hid his thoughts. So that one day over the inevitable cup of coffee a quiet, flat statement came out. I was dumbfounded: "Ruby, I have got to go to South America!"

I sat frozen to the seat, just staring at him:

"Now, darling girl," he rushed on, "don't you worry, I've got it all worked out – South America's a land of endless opportunities – you haven't a *thing* to worry about. I'll get a job straight away and before you know it, you'll be on your way out to join me. We'll get married out there."

I blinked hard; "B-but w-what about your m-medical career?"

He shrugged resignedly; "Just have to give the idea up, not enough money. Can't think what's gone wrong but seems there's been a mix-up somewhere. It'll take ages to get a reply from China. No, there's nothing for it I'm afraid, I'll have to give up the idea."

Then out came a resumé of the plans. He was going with another medical student named Lennie, who it appeared was avid for adventure in the golden land. Both were supremely optimistic, quite convinced that they would soon make a fortune in South America. After paying ten pounds for steerage accommodation on the R.M.S. *Orita*, they each had twenty pounds in their pocket to face the unknown country. I at that time still full of apprehension about white slavers and other evil-doers in general stitched a strong calico body-belt with a pocket in which to store the precious pounds, and this Jim solemnly promised to wear at all times. And so another tearful farewell, this time alone at the flat where we spent the last few hours playing despairing music, all in a minor key which in no way helped either of us.

No-one at hospital knew about all this until the absence of the two students at lectures gave rise to wild rumours which swept through the medical school and among the nurses. These romance-starved girls kept a keen eye on our notice board where all our letters were posted and when letters for me arrived from such ports as La Rochelle, Coruña, Vigo, and Rio de Janeiro, many curious glances were shot at me with a rather wistful expression indicating their hope that I would tell them all about it. I kept my own counsel with the exception of Rene and Husky, who of course knew all about it.

Jimmy's fluent pen gave wings to my imagination:

Through his eyes I saw the filthy conditions under which they were travelling – three hundred steerage passengers packed like sardines in a tin. Curiosity was rife among the first and second class passengers as to why the two obviously well-educated Englishmen were travelling rough – it was agreed the answer must be to see life in the raw to gather material for novels. The two men picked up a smattering of Spanish from their fellow passengers all of whom were nationals of South America.

After disembarkation at Montevideo, I received a very long letter relating all the happenings of their first thirty-six hours in port, and the manner in which they found a job. Studying an armful of papers, all in Spanish, they came across the heading, 'Ferrocarril Central del Uruguay', the railways of the country, and underneath an English-sounding address, this they thought was their best bet. And so, the following morning, each dressed in his one and only suit, complete with their university tie puffed out conspicuously, and calling-card, they set out to try and find the Head Office with the aid of Hugo's Spanish Phrase Book. The search ended at an imposing-looking building. They were greeted courteously in the outer office by the Spanish clerk, in his own language. With a grand flourish they presented their card and asked to see the manager:

The clerk answered politely in English:

"Señors, please to be seated. I shall ascertain if Mr. F. is at liberty to see you; if he is not I shall myself for you make the appointment." He half-bowed and left the room; soon to return:

"The manager is for the moment, free . . . Please to follow me, Señors."

He led them into a large, luxurious office where they found the general manager of the Ferrocarril Central del Uruguay Company seated behind an enormous desk smoking a large cigar. He was obviously

Cambridge English and *very* polite, stating that he was "simply charmed" to welcome two of his countrymen to Montevideo. And then proceeded, in the manner of all Englishmen abroad to talk about the weather, followed by sports, chiefly rugger, and ending with travel. It appeared that the manager's opinion of these two young unexpected visitors was similar to those on board ship – obviously on a sight-seeing tour, gathering material for a book – no doubt wealthy. He intimated how fortunate they were and what a splendid thing it was to see the world when young; he carefully lit another cigar and leaned back in his comfortable swing chair, blew out rings of fragrant smoke and enquired congenially:

"Well, gentlemen, and what may I do for you?"

"We want a job!" they stated in chorus.

Mr. F. stared at them, his eyes lingering a moment on the university ties; "I *beg* your pardon!"

"We need a job!"

The general manager of the Ferrocarril Central del Uruguay stiffened and carefully flicked off the ash from his cigar, then remarked coldly:

"Do you mean to tell me that you two young men have come out from England, walked into my office and had the audacity to expect me to give you a job!" He drew hard on his cigar. "I am forced to conclude that you are in need of money! I regret that I must inform you that all – and I repeat, all – our British employees are interviewed in London."

Lennie smiled apologetically, then said coaxingly:

"But Sir, we are willing to do anything, go anywhere . . ." and added shrewdly, "if you employ us, sir, it will save the company two passages out!"

Mr. F. sat quietly summing up his visitors . . . Suddenly, he gave a chuckle; "Never heard of before . . . *Most* unusual . . . I shall have to think about it . . . meanwhile, gentlemen, I shall be glad if you will be my guests this evening at the British Club. I'm quite sure that my wife will wish you to join us at dinner . . . Shall we say then at seven at the club?" He gave them directions how to find it.

The invitation was accepted with delight.

The evening ended after an excellent dinner at the manager's palatial home. While bidding them 'good-night' he told them to present themselves at his office at precisely ten o'clock in the morning. The interview ended by Jim being sent to the station north at Rivera on the border of Brazil, within a few paces of the Santayana. Lennie was posted at Timeranbuco, about a hundred miles south. Only Spanish was spoken at these remote outposts, and in the station office nothing but Spanish was spoken, so they soon learned the musical, flowery language.

From the frequent letters I gleaned masses of information about the country to which I was supposed to travel just as soon as Jim had saved up the passage money. It sounded to me a mixture of paradise and purgatory . . . 'Imagine', wrote Jim, 'a day twice as hot as any you've known in an English summer. It is not too uncomfortable at the moment for it's the so-called cool, dry season. At night the breeze is cool and the sky as light as day – but with a purple light if there is a moon. Imagine crooning, whispering, buzzing – all the bustle of a myriad life around you. At night the songsters awake; human, bird and beast. Guitars and tangos; love calls and quaint bird-song mingled with the harsh croak of frogs and the screams of animals. In fact everything that can make a noise, augments a hymn of thankfulness for the coolness of the night.

'Flowers literally in profusion, roses all the year round, and honeysuckle. The incredibly numerous varieties of simply marvellous wild flowers of beautiful, if bizarre colours, absolutely stagger one. The day is hard, the night wonderful!'

And the harsh side of the tropical paradise:

'. . . It appears that during the day man has to fight myriads of smaller beasties merely for the privilege of living; mosquitoes, flies; ants of every conceivable shape and colour, and every insect, microbe and parasite that crawls, flies, hops, stings, bites and even pinches!'

It seemed to me that if one was prepared to put up with appalling heat, dirt, ignorance and laziness of the local people, there were a variety of ways in which to get rich quickly, that is if one were gifted with a keen business sense. In the reputed 'them thar hills' it was whispered gold was to be found, as yet untouched. On the various types of ranches too were other sources of wealth.

The trouble was I felt convinced that neither Jim nor myself had any business sense at all. It worried me too that he had given up medicine; for although I still found some aspects of nursing repulsive it was undeniable that I found great joy in being able to relieve pain, even in a small way. And so when his letter came urging both Rene and myself to come out to Buenos Aires, where he'd found a job for us at the Anglo-American hospital, I thought the matter through to the firm conclusion that I would allow *nothing* to persuade me to leave England until I was fully qualified as a nurse. I was just as sure that Jimmy would never find happiness in pursuing gold.

Meanwhile fate or providence – was quietly conspiring to bring my impulsive fiancé back to England, for quite suddenly and unexpectedly, money became available for him to carry on with medicine. This exciting news came to me from a Dymond relative, worded a little vaguely, but begging me to get in touch with Jim and beg him to come home. I wrote a letter and as week after week passed with no reply, I was flung into a state of restless anxiety . . . I waited and waited, but nothing came.

Then some weeks later when I was on night duty and giving out the ten o'clock medicines the ward phone rang. I lifted the receiver.

"Nurse Morris?" queried Curly, the night-porter.

"Speaking . . ." and waited to be informed of an emergency.

"Half a mo' . . ."

"Hello, Ruby!" said the cool, calm voice of Jimmy.

I nearly dropped with fright, then I whispered idiotically, "Is it you?"

"Just got back this morning," he said, for all the world as though he'd been away for a long weekend, "Any hope of seeing you in the morning?"

"Yes, it's my morning off."

"The usual place, O.K.?"

Throughout the night my heart jumped all over the place torn by conflicting emotions. Thrilled, shy, excited and terrified. I left Norfolk Square in the morning feeling exhausted and as remote as the Himalayas. But at the sight of the tall, handsome figure bronzed by the tropical sun, all my fears evaporated . . . and within minutes it really did seem as though he'd only been away for a weekend. We left the Blue Cat and sauntered along to our seat by Peter Pan, and there with hands clasped we talked over the problems of the immediate future. It turned out that the windfall of money was a mere eighty-five pounds which had to cover all expenses and examination fees, and keep him until he was qualified. There was no hope for a penny more. He patted my hand; "Now, Ruby dear, don't you worry, I've got it all worked out. It's not quite as grim as it sounds. I can get all the medical books with the money I saved for your passage out, and I saved my passage home too – took a heck of a time finding a ship I can tell you . . . Gosh, the *sacks* of potatoes I peeled! I'm seeing the Dean this afternoon to ask if I can sit for L.M.S.S.A. next July, and Conjoint in October . . . But lummy, I'll just have to get through the lot at first go, or I'm completely sunk."

It was my turn to pat his hand; "You will, I'm sure you will, darling."

"By golly, I hope you're right, it's not going to be easy."

I was still missing my two friends – Rene was now with Mrs. Coward's Co-op of private nurses, and Husky was a sister at Miss Simpson's Surgical and Maternity Nursing Home in Welbeck Street. I too had got through all my exams and now had the Hospital and State Certificates, but now I was working out my months of sick leave. It was late autumn and all too soon it was my turn to pack my bags and go to the East End Maternity Hospital to do my midwifery training.

In those days of the 'twenties midwifery training was a gruelling six months, long hours, snatched sleep and study in off-duty times. Our times off were short and meant there was little chance for Jim and I to meet, so once more the pen came into its own. Soon he was telling me on paper about an idea his friend, George Carnegie Brown, another student trying to stretch sixpence into a pound, had put to him, which was an invitation to share the flat he'd found in Marylebone, and so halve expenses. Both shared another distress – they were in love. George had lost his heart to a junior nurse, Pat Wymer, a tall attractive blue-eyed girl. It was a good idea and he accepted it.

I had dreaded going to the East End being convinced I would loathe it, because of the shock I had when I first went to St. Mary's. I was nineteen and on my second ward when one quiet afternoon a nurse came rushing in with a note from her labour-ward Sister, requesting to borrow a nurse for a few hours as they were frantically busy and a difficult case was in progress. I was sent and arrived in the labour-ward sweating with fear. I had never seen a birth, either human or animal, and my knowledge of anatomy at that time was practically nil. The sight that met my eyes did me more harm than what was happening to the patient, for she mercifully was lightly under an anaesthetic; she was a high-forceps delivery. Sheer will-power prevented me from screaming and running out of the labour-ward and from the hospital for ever.

And on that occasion instead of holding back an arm as in the 'Ku Klux Klan fashion', I now had to hold onto a leg; I swayed dangerously in a near faint but was wrenched back to the troubled world by the patient who started shouting:

"Aw, aw, Gawd save us . . . Just you wite till I kin lay me 'ands on yer our 'arry. I'll give yer wot for . . . Aw, aw, I tell yer I don't want this dratted biby . . . don't want it . . . Aw, Gawd save us . . ." The nurse at her head quickly poured onto the face mask, more chloroform and the shouting stopped.

Glamour was not added to love's young dream:

But in spite of my loathing, to my surprise it was at midwifery I achieved my shining hour. For some reason I found I had a similar influence over a woman in labour as I had with hysterical patients. More surprising still, theory presented no problem. I became very attached to the patients who showed so much concern about the over-worked nurses.

They did all they could to save us unnecessary running about. When Sister was off-duty they'd sing out:

"Blimey, ducks, yer look that tired, sit *down.* Cum on now, tike the wite offof yer feet . . . Sit down, Sister ain't abart . . . 'ere give me the little tike, I kin manage 'im . . ."

This from women whose whole life was one unending round of drudgery, and for whom having a baby in the hospital was the only rest and holiday they were ever likely to get. The shabby hospital dressing gowns were pathetically worn in the small of the back by the constant rubbings to try and ease the pain. In those days it was seldom that the poor knew the luxury of an anaesthetic. They were given only in cases of extreme necessity. Our rota system of calls to the labour-ward was such that often the same nurse would find herself called up three nights running. We were not allowed time off to make up for lost sleep, and all too often we worked in a daze of fatigue.

Jimmy was doing his 'midder' course at Queen Charlotte's Hospital and so his hours too were uncertain. But his letters sustained me through the long hours and gave me an incentive to stay awake during our lectures from Dr. Oxley, the hospital's obstetrician. Five long weeks passed before we were able to meet, and a sentence in Jim's letter hit me with a stab of anxiety; '. . . When we meet on Friday, there's something I want to talk over with you . . .'

When we met outside Piccadilly Corner House he was looking as tired as I felt, but there was a sense of repressed excitement in him; "Let's have tea first, darling, then we'll go along to the gardens," he said tucking my arm in his. But later sitting in the autumn sunshine with birds chirping merrily nearby, my heart dropped with a thud when my lover suddenly said after a long pause: "Lummy, I feel so nervous . . . I'm scared stiff!"

He's off to Timbuktu, I thought miserably. I braced myself for the coming shock and asked quietly:

"Now, my dear, tell me what's gone wrong?"

He fidgeted about restlessly, took ages it seemed in lighting a cigarette. Then he took my hand and looked down at me with a most solemn expression:

"Dearest girl . . . I-I've been thinking . . . I'm absolutely fed up with only cafes to go to, and taking bus rides . . . Darling girl . . . Let's get married!"

Dumbfounded, I just sat and stared at him:

"Married! Get married! Us!"

He grinned adorably, "Well, why not? People do, you know!"

"B-but we *can't* – we're not qualified – we've no money – we agreed to wait two years before even thinking of it!" I rattled off the facts, "And besides I'll be sent home in disgrace . . . It's the strictest rule you know."

He grinned again impishly, "They won't find out, we'll keep it a dark secret. Now I can tell you another secret *and* a bit of good news." He paused so long I broke out irritably:

"Oh, for heaven's sake, go *on* . . . What *is* it?"

"George and Pat have!"

"Have *what*?"

"Got married," said he triumphantly.

"Pat!" my junior a married woman! "But how, when?"

"A few weeks ago at a registry office, only knew myself a couple of days ago . . ." he went on eagerly, "They're terribly keen for us to get married . . . What do you think? Please, *please* say yes."

I gazed away into space, lost in thought . . . The idea appalled me – a secret marriage! No chapel, no orange blossom, no white wedding . . . A secret marriage from the East End:

I protested feebly, "But how about money?"

"Money! Oh, dear, oh dear," he teased, "what *can* we do about that!" then drew out from his pocket a slip of paper and waved it at me, "Look, my little love . . . From my wonderful Dad in Yunnan."

It was a cheque for fifty pounds!

I gazed at this fortune spellbound. Then suddenly the idea of getting married in a 'Gretna Green' fashion seemed wildly romantic and exciting. It had other advantages too; in keeping with our horror of ever being under an obligation to people, this would mean no-one would be put to inconvenience or expense. More important it would prove our love and faith in each other. So I said, "Oh, yes, let's do it, let's get married!"

Then Jimmy cried out to the birds, trees and sky: "There now . . . Oh, boy, oh boy, ain't life *wonderful,* ain't life *great*." I found myself enveloped in strong arms, then three heartbeats later he was saying: "I tell you what we'll do, we'll keep most of Dad's cheque then when we're qualified we'll go on our honeymoon!"

I went back to the East End with feathers in my brain and tremors in my heart. For by now I had learned that Elmslie Dymond was a man of action.

Sure enough a week later along came a letter:

". . . It's all settled, my darling, the blessèd moment that will link us for ever is fixed for Saturday, 6th December, 2.30 p.m. at the Paddington Registry Office. Pat will meet you outside St. Mary's, and George and Rene will sign as witnesses . . . I'll leave it up to you to demand your half-day off, and also arrange things with Husky and Rene!"

To demand anything of a matron was to court instant refusal, and so making an effort to quieten my fluttering heart and with Jim's letter tucked inside my uniform I trotted down to her office. Matron Anderson, a Scot and a wonderful woman, was seated at her desk writing:

"Good-morning, Matron," I began in what I hoped was a voice full of confidence: "Matron, please may I arrange to take my half-day off on Saturday, December 6th . . . and er . . . may I go off duty at twelve? You see it's imperative for me to be down in the West End by two-thirty . . ." A sudden brain-wave made me add, "I have to attend a most important committee meeting!"

What she thought of that unlikely committee meeting I shall never know; but she cheerfully waved me away; "Och, and away wi ye, Nurse Morris, don't come bothering me with sich silly little requests. If it's convenient for your labour-ward Sister to let you go, you may do so, but if it's not, then of course you can't."

"Thank you, Matron, I understand. Good-morning."

I fled upstairs and found the labour-ward Sister:

"Please, Sister, Matron says I'm to be allowed off duty at twelve sharp on Saturday, 6th . . . You see I simply have to be down at the West End by half-past two."

She replied casually: "That will be all right, Nurse, providing you're not on a case. Naturally, if you are then you'll have to stay on to clear up."

"Yes, Sister, of course, Sister. Thank you, Sister."

And to my faithful 'musketeers' I wrote hasty notes, and in a matter of hours got their replies both worded to the effect that – come hell or high water, they would 'wangle' their off-duty. Rene added the postscript; "Ruby love, we're going shopping! Let me know when you can get off, we'll meet outside Swan and Edgar's."

Chapter Nineteen

It was a cold, raw morning, that morning of 6th December, 1929, when I wakened with an alarming sense of impending illness – there was a strange tightness in my chest. I sat up in bed with tousled hair, still half asleep; "*Now* what's the matter with me!" I muttered, as I struggled out of bed to go and have a diagnostic look in the mirror . . . Dreadful sight! A quick mind-probing gave me the answer. I was conscience-stricken knowing that for the first time in my life I had not confided in my beloved brother George, nor with my two other close friends, Bill and Cliff. But the pangs vanished with the arrival of a letter from Jimmy – the most precious I'd ever received. Before going down to breakfast I peeped into my wardrobe and surveyed the result of my shopping spree with Rene, her gifts to me. There they were – the new pale blue coat and stylish white dress, and a rather perky little hat – sure proof that this was my wedding day.

I crossed my fingers; "Will our luck hold, I wonder . . . *will* it . . . Oh, dear, what if we both have a case! Maybe I won't be married after all!" I closed the cupboard and hurried down to breakfast. And when I tripped upstairs to my ward the night nurse called out to me cheerily: "Got a case for you, Morris, she's in the waiting room . . ." I went in with leaden feet, and found a young fragile looking girl: "Hello, dear," said I brightly and hopefully, "Your pains are getting *much* stronger now, aren't they?"

She sniffed, "No, they ain't, Nurse, just niggling, that's wot they are – ever so trying it is!"

I reached for the dressing-gown; "Well now," I said briskly, "come along, there's a good girl – get up, it's so much quicker if you keep on moving about."

Fortunately for the girl and for me the baby was in as great a hurry to get into the world as I was to get off-duty. Without fuss or bother it emerged and yelled lustily, early enough for me to clear up and leave the labour-ward spotless for the next case. I dashed up to my room at twelve-fifteen, flung off my uniform; in and out of the bath in a jiffy, then at last donned in the new outfit I climbed onto a chair to see the full-length result – for we had no long mirror in our room . . .

"Umm . . . not too bad," said Martha to Ruby. With Ruby uppermost and winged feet I rushed down the stairs, out of the front door which slammed with a bang behind me . . . I was on my way to be married! A wave of Celtic emotion swept through me as I ran at full-speed to catch the oncoming bus.

Having eaten almost nothing at breakfast I arrived at Paddington Underground feeling rather light-headed. Outside St. Mary's I found a very agitated Pat waiting for me; "Oh, *Ruby,* thank *goodness* you've come – I've been on pins, thought you must be on a bad case . . ."

"I *was* on a case . . ." I puffed.

"Gosh, you're as pale as a ghost . . ." she took my arm and gave it an assuring little squeeze. "There's nothing to be scared about, honestly love, it's quite easy . . . George and I are so thrilled about it."

At the registry office there stood Rene, Husky, and George Brown, with Jimmy in the centre looking pale but distinguished in the brand new suit hired from Moss Bros. The proceedings that followed are a blur in my memory, but one stands out in vivid colour – the Registrar himself, who looked exactly like an undertaker. A cadaverous man of medium height in a black suit, long pale narrow face topped by a scrawny neck encircled by a high, stiff white collar, pinze-nez perched on the pinched, red-tipped nose from the end of which a drop of moisture hung precariously – the sight of it fascinated me – would it, or would it not, stay there!

The marriage lines were intoned in sepulchral voice, I remember murmuring "Yes," here and there, and "I do", then the cold shock of the gold ring being slipped on to my finger. The Registrar handed Jim the marriage certificate, gave us a wintry smile and wished us great happiness. With all the formalities over, Mr. and Mrs. E. C. Dymond walked out into the bitter cold of winter, with Spring in their heart and hopes for the future . . . I was a married woman . . . Due back on duty by ten o'clock. The celebration meal of course was on the second floor of the Piccadilly Corner House. We were shown to our booked table while the orchestra was most suitably playing "Danny Boy" . . . The tension was over and we felt completely carefree.

At nine o'clock we trooped out again in the cold and frosty air, and on down into the Underground. Kisses and hugs all round as the train came thundering in . . . Jim held me close and whispered:

"Goodnight, my darling little wife . . . Now you are all mine, just you watch me fight for *us.*"

Before going back into hospital I took off my wedding ring and tied it onto a ribbon and hung it round my neck. The minute my head touched the pillow I fell into an exhausted sleep . . . Only to be woken at midnight with a loud knock at my door:

"Nurse Morris . . . Quickly . . . An urgent case." Which ended at dawn.

For the last two months of our training we nurses worked on 'District' during which time we were obliged to fill our case books with a minimum of fifty deliveries. All nurses dreaded their first call-out to a case, and I was no exception. Delivering a baby in a hospital with the aid of Sister, and an obstetrician on call should anything go wrong, was one thing. But alone, armed with only a midwife's bag, was quite another. My first call-out came on a bitter star-lit night at two o'clock. From the first urgent knock at our door we were allowed only three minutes to be up, dressed and outside ready to follow the escort who came for us.

My escort that night was a very tall, gangling length of man who informed me dourly: "We'll 'ave ter 'urry, Nurse. Missis was far on when I left the 'ouse." He set off at such a pace I had to run to keep up with him. "Is this a first baby?" I puffed out anxiously:

"Blimey, no," he snorted gloomily, "anythin' but . . . it's the sixteenth!"

I flung up a short prayer to the starry heavens; "Please, oh, please let the baby be safely there before we get there!"

I found my prayer answered for on arrival at the tenement hovel, I was greeted cheerfully by a very fat woman laying in a big bed in the tiny room; "Hello, love, yer too lite – 'e's just popped out, 'e's *that* bonny . . ." the expectant father dumped my bag and promptly disappeared. I drew back the grubby bed-sheet and there lay a very large baby boy contentedly sucking his thumb. She mistook my look of relief for that of concern for she added encouragingly: "There now, ducks, don't take on so, it weren't your fault . . . yer've still got the afterbirth ter do."

There seemed to be swarms of children about all interested in what was happening to Mum, for small heads kept on peering round the door. I shooed them all away and got on with the job. An aged crone shuffled in carrying a kettle of hot water, and an armful of newspapers. This was all I had to cope with the situation.

We always called on our cases for ten days after the birth, bathing the baby and the mother. I came to know and love the East End cockneys, unbeaten anywhere in the world for their good humour and generosity.

An example of their kindness was shown on my first visit to my first case, the mother of sixteen. She probed about under her pillow and brought out a tattered brown paper parcel:

"This 'ere is for you, Nurse," she beamed at me, "Last night I says to our Gert, I says, 'That there little nurse looked that perishing cold last night, jist you go on art and get 'er something', it's fer you ducks ter keep you warm."

I opened the parcel and out came two cylinder lengths of deep cream wool material, and yards of shocking purple lace; "I'll mike a luvly vest fer yer, ducky," said my patient, well pleased, "All yer need ter do is stitch up top and bottom and tack on the lace – it'll keep yer that cosy."

The following day I received a pair of bright green garters, decorated with pink rosettes; I felt so touched I kept them for years.

By May I was in a state of frantic swotting for the Maternity and C.M.B. exams; then one afternoon just as I'd got myself deep in reciting aloud the various positions of 'baby' in relation to mother, Husky most unexpectedly burst into my room; "News, news, news!" she proclaimed gaily. I got up yawning widely with my book clasped to my bosom; "Hello, Husky bach, lovely to see you but what's the news?"

With great deliberation she delayed answering by picking up this and that, including taking my medical book by saying: "Here, give me that 'thriller' you're reading, and *sit down*."

I sat down and picked up another tome which I raised threateningly:

"Tell me, tell me, tell me . . . or else!"

She cocked her head on one side, paused then announced casually:

"How would you like to work with me at Welbeck Street?"

I leapt to my feet as though shot from a gun:

"How would I *like*! Oh, you can't mean it, are you pulling my leg?"

"I'm certainly not, Ruby Morris – Sorry, Dymond . . . There's a vacancy coming up soon and Miss Simpson asked me yesterday if I knew a St. Mary's trained nurse – she's got a thing about Mary's – so of course I said at once that my friend was due to take her 'midder' exams next week. She told me to book you! You'll be having the room next to mine at our quarters in Blandlord Street."

I flung myself into her arms and almost cried with joy, until I remembered the formidable exams: "Oh, what marvellous luck, but Husky, what if I don't pass! Oh, dear, what if I don't pass!"

"Calm down," said my friend, "Calm down . . . Just don't panic that's all . . . You'll pass, I've always told you you know more than you think . . . By the way this will mean that you and Jim will be able to meet more often – I'll scout around and see if I can find a flat or something near Welbeck Street . . . But my goodness you'll have to be jolly careful not to let your secret out. If Miss Simpson finds out you're married, bang goes your job!"

And *that* was the beginning of my shining hour:

To be offered a post as Sister at the then London's leading Nursing Home was just wonderful luck. And the highlight of it all came on the morning when I was summoned to Matron's office to hear the result of my exams. I presented myself there in spotless uniform and stood with damp hands clasped behind my back waiting for the axe to fall. But both Matron and Dr. Oxley were smiling up at me kindly:

"Good morning, Nurse Morris – and congratulations!"

The miracle of the age – I had passed both parts of the exam with high marks. I relaxed and made an effort of will not to burst into sobs of relief. Matron said, "I think you do know, Nurse, that District Sister Jenner has been ill and is to take six months sick leave. Dr. Oxley and I would like you to take her place until she comes back."

I felt quite stunned and went fiery hot all over.

This too was a thrilling compliment, to be offered the post of District Sister immediately after qualifying. But the awful moment had now come when I had to confess my marriage. I fidgeted, stammered and choked. They both regarded me kindly giving me time to pull myself together. My Maternity and C.M.B. Certificates were on the desk before Dr. Oxley. He took up his pen and asked for my second name.

I took in a deep breath and gasped: "Please Sir, will you write Dymond instead of Morris as my surname!"

There was a sudden shocked silence. Both heads shot up with a jerk. They just sat and stared at me. I said, "Well, you s-see," and went on in a small voice, "You see . . . I-I'm m-married . . ."

It was Matron who spoke first: "Well, upon my soul! D'ye hear the like of that, Dr. Oxley? Why, bless my soul, what *are* the young coming to these days!" She fell silent for a long moment, ruminating, then she looked at me with a twinkle in her eye:

"Tell me, Nurse, did this happy event take place on the day of that 'important' committee meeting?"

I blushed scarlet: "Yes, Matron . . . I'm sorry, Matron . . ."

But Dr. Oxley threw back his head and roared with laughter: "Well, I must say we've a real little dark horse here, eh, Matron?" Once more he took up his pen, "Now, Nurse, tell me exactly how I'm to sign these certificates?"

"My name is Ruby Margaretta Dymond, Sir."

"I take it you wish Matron and me to keep your secret?"

"Oh, yes, indeed *please*, sir, I simply have to have a job until my husband qualifies . . . he hopes to get L.M.S.S.A. in July and Conjoint in October."

Dr. Oxley raised an eyebrow: "By jove . . . L.M.S.S.A. *and* Conjoint in October . . . Umm, that's what I call being heroic . . . Don't worry, Nurse, we'll keep your secret . . . Now how about being District Sister for us?"

So I stumbled on to explain why I couldn't accept the post: "Well, Nurse," Dr. Oxley said kindly; "Well, we have to congratulate you on that too, but we'll be very sorry to lose you. But look here now we can't have a hospital romance right under our noses and not meet your husband, can we? Is he coming here to take you to the West End?"

"Yes, Sir, he is."

When Jimmy arrived I first introduced him to some of the student nurses as my fiancé. Later in Matron's office I felt *quite* three inches taller when Dr. Oxley remarked: "We are very sorry indeed to lose her, Mr. Dymond, she's a splendid midwife. By the way, jolly good luck to you in your exams."

And so from the rag, tag and bobtail of the East End, I went straight to the silks and satins of the West End. Very fortunately for me Miss Simpson took me on the strength of Husky's recommendation, and at my interview with her she did not bother to ask to see my certificates. I was soon settled in my new quarters in Blandford Street, and shortly afterwards my wonderful Husky came bounding into my room: "Got something for Jim," said she beaming like a fond mother, "a room with its own bathroom – an annexe in a private house in Baker Street. Here's the address, tell Jim to get along there as soon as he can, or he may miss it. It's got a lovely view of the park."

So he too was soon installed in what was our first 'home'. Of course I could not stay there, but all my off-duty times I threw off being Nurse Martha and became Ruby Dymond – wife.

And at St. Mary's, Elmslie Chalmers Dymond became something of a mystery man, more absent than present, seldom turning up for lectures, much to the scathing disgust of his lecturers! He confided in no one, only I knew of the intensive study that was going on, only I saw the tall hunched figure bowed over a mountain of books on the table near the window, and masses of writing paper – heavy tomes on Medicine, Midwifery and Gynaecology; Materia Medica and Pharmacology . . . writing, writing, writing . . . taking down copious meticulous notes in small neat handwriting; endless sketches of anatomy . . . absorbing masses of knowledge.

Jim Dymond's method of concentrating was to have his small crystal-wireless set on at full blast. It was on morning, noon and night. The moment he became aware of it he knew he'd lost concentration. So up to pace the floor, wash hands and face in cold water; drink mugs of black coffee, then back to the grind. This went on until the eve of 24th July, 1931, the day before sitting for the L.M.S.S.A.

All during this time he had been like a man training for the priesthood; a person in retreat, a man obsessed. My nervousness showed itself like a storm-tossed sea, all raging within. While his was always silent and ice-cold calm.

At St. Mary's there were snorts of derision among the medical students; "Quite honestly, old man, the chap hasn't a hope of passing *anything* . . . As for having a crack at Conjoint, it's enough to make a cat laugh."

"Couldn't agree more," said another, "Imagine the nerve of the fellow having a go at the whole lot!"

But Curly, on duty at the lodge, overheard these remarks being nearby a group of students, broke in, his faith in his hero was absolute: "Don't you be so sure, cock," said he, "There's more to that there Mr. Dymond than meets the eye – I'd take a bet on him passing any day!"

This remark set the ball rolling, and a spate of heavy betting was on – with the odds stacked high against the enigmatic Dymond.

Chapter Twenty

Curly later reported to Jim the happenings of the day when the L.M.S.S.A. examination results were posted up on the board. Excited groups of students gathered round the board obviously mentally adding up their bets. The murmurings died away into silence as they saw that Elmslie Chalmers Dymond had passed in all subjects with top marks. Presently Curly had strolled back to the lodge whistling while the coins in his pockets made a merry jingle. The newly qualified Dr. E. C. Dymond promptly took a two-weeks locum at the Paddington Infirmary. He was greatly elated at the thought of his first earnings – eight guineas . . . Oh, the things we were going to do with that money! Even a quarter would have cost twice as much.

I happened to be off-duty on his pay-day and when I came into our room he greeted me with a shy smile. I expected him to produce the eight pounds with a proud smile, counting them out one by one. Instead he took from his pocket a tiny parcel, then with his wonderful smile he held it out to me; "It's for you, darling . . . I've had this 'cooked-up' for a long time."

I opened it and there on its cushion of black velvet lay the daintiest diamond ring I'd ever seen! A lump came into my throat . . . It seemed to me the sparkle from the diamonds emanated rays of poignant love . . . I'd just become engaged! I flung myself into my husband's arms and wept. After seven months of marriage I'd become engaged.

Then came the second round of hard grind, the advanced repetition of the same subjects – on which he'd just been examined – to be ready for Conjoint in October. I was very happy in my work at Welbeck Street. Miss Simpson and the staff Sisters were very friendly and jolly people, and it was sheer joy working with Husky.

Life settled down into its usual pattern of silence in our room, the only difference being that it was more intense. Thus when sitting opposite my husband I took to day-dreaming. I gazed out of the window, watched the clouds flying by, and listened to the ducks quacking and splashing about on the pond in the park. But more and more I found my attention being drawn back into the room and on to the mantelshelf where there was a growing pile of letters from China. Every time I saw the foreign stamp on a letter dropped on the mat in the tiny hall, I felt a quick stab of anxiety . . . China!

The word seemed to hover in the air although we did not talk about it. It went without saying that the immediate urgency was to pass Conjoint. But my intuition was hard at work. I knew that the day would come when I would have to make a decision about the country to which, as a child, I'd sworn never to go.

In the silences I thought over the implications contained in those letters. No-one said in so many words 'It is your duty to come back to China', but instead kept on giving vivid descriptions of the conditions out there, of the urgent need for Western medicine and Western drugs. And too there was the task of the problems of obscure and loathsome diseases; of the fight against the slavery of young girls; the rescue of the surplus girl-babies who were thrown to the wolves outside city gates. All this, and more besides slowly ate into my mind like a burrowing worm.

Later, I found myself rehearsing a new role for myself:

Staunch young wife quietly prepares to follow noble husband to the uttermost ends of the earth . . . Visions appeared before my inner eye . . . A tall, thin doctor – this man before me who almost always was completely oblivious of my presence – This doctor bending over a rickety operating-table absorbed in doing delicate operations by hurricane lamps or candlelight. The tall man being borne along on the shoulder of four rickshaw coolies bearing a sedan chair up high mountains to reach desperately sick people, or answering a call from a wealthy Mandarin. Saw him coping with cholera epidemics, smallpox and leprosy . . . But the mere word brought the visions to a sudden stop . . . I'd *seen* pictures of the ravages of the disease in Jimmy's medical books! . . . Oh, no, *no*, I could *never* go there.

So by the time it was October we were both worn out and on edge. Jim seemed drained of vitality and he'd lost a lot of weight. He was so mentally fatigued I was afraid his mind would go blank at some crucial questions, as mine was so apt to do.

Again the betting game at hospital was in full swing:

Dymond just could *not* pull it off again. More than ever he'd been the invisible man, so with the exception of Curly and a few other brave souls the betting was still heavily against his chances.

On the first day of the written exams it was my day off. Jimmy was weary to the extent of indifference as to the outcome; I suffered enough quakes for the two of us. Each day when I enquired how it had gone he replied dully: "Haven't a clue . . . Just wrote down all I knew, got up and left the room. Felt a awful ass as I seemed to be the first out each time, and the chaps started stamping their feet." On the last morning I was there too to wish him good-luck. He looked deathly pale, and as soon as he'd gone I started my usual pacing the floor and sudden departures to the bathroom.

And in twenty minutes he rushed back into the room like an agitated whirlwind: "My card! My card! Can't find it, it's not on me. Where is it? Have *you* got it!" A frantic search for Card 213 without which he would not be allowed into the examination room . . . Ah, there it was – in the pocket of his dressing-gown.

This time I went to meet him:

As usual, he was the first out:

"How did you go on, darling?"

"Haven't a clue!"

"Decent questions?"

"Not too bad . . . Oh, heck, let's go and have coffee!"

On the first day of the ten-day holiday due to me Jimmy received the results of the exams. He came back from St. Mary's and tore into our room with dynamic energy; I was swept up into his arms:

"Oh, ain't life wonderful, ain't life simply *great*! It's all over, darling, all the tension and worry's over . . . I've passed the lot!" He'd got top marks in most, excelling in Midwifery and Gynaecology.

So Dymond had pulled it off again and once more Curly's pockets tinkled. And at long last we went off to Clevedon for that belated honeymoon, which like most honeymoons turned out to be a mixture of pathos and comedy. When we got back to Baker Street Jim picked up the solitary envelope lying on the mat, glanced casually at it, saying: "Looks like a hospital circular," and tossed it on to the table, "I'll make us some tea . . ."

Presently as we sipped it in what by now had become a habit, complete silence, Jim reached out for a biscuit, then idly picked up the letter, and I went off into thoughts of my own. Grateful thoughts about my family and friends who had borne no resentment at our getting married in secret. I was especially relieved about George, the one who felt it most, but his nature is such that he's incapable of harbouring resentment against anyone. And then too . . . But a sudden loud exclamation from Jimmy brought me back with a jerk:

"Lummy!" he was staring at the letter as though fascinated.

"Whatever's wrong darling?" my heart thumped and turned over.

"Oh, lummy!" he responded with his favourite slang word.

"For heaven's sake – *what is it*?"

"A JOB."

"Where!"

"China! On the South coast . . . A HOSPITAL."

"When?"

"Just as soon as we can get there . . . Seems they're desperately over-worked! Passages paid . . . Kit and household allowance."

A long, long silence.

Then in a quiet, tight voice, my husband said: "Well, Ruby, what is the answer?"

Once more those pleading blue-grey eyes!

It was more than anyone could bear, and I thought . . . your rehearsal's over . . . the curtain's up . . . Staunch little wife walks onto stage; while aloud I said:

"Yes, of *course*, Jimmy bach," Celtic emotion flooded my being, "Of course, dearest, if you want to go to China – then so do I."

The next few weeks found us rushing hither and thither in a state of turmoil. I resigned my post at Welbeck Street, and we spent days in frantic shopping. Then came the day when we had to have anti-cholera and typhoid injections. And within hours both of us lay prone on our respective beds, racked with fever, aching joints and raging heads. On the second evening of misery, our ministering angel, Marie Huskinson turned up unexpectedly, her arms laden with bags of fruit and a bottle of Eau-de-Cologne.

She bathed our fevered brows remarking with impish grin:

"Well, if you two darlings insist on going off to the other ends of the earth, you must expect to suffer. This is only the *beginning,* you know!"

But by the time she'd made our beds, fed us with soup and toast, keeping up a patter of her nonsense rhymes, we were laughing and knew that after all, death was not at hand.

Although she bantered light-heartedly, she, Bill and Cliff took a very dim view of our going to China; not so Rene who was thrilled: "Who knows, Ruby love, one day I may come out and visit you in China!"

When I had a few breathing spells from rushing about I sat before our gas-fire building up pictures of the wonderful ship on which we should travel. I remembered those glorious vessels in Liverpool on which I had been so sure I would travel. Of *course* it would be huge with *three* funnels and freshly painted.

The day of embarkation dawned, dark, cold and overcast; I was seething with excitement. We checked everything – passports, luggage clearly labelled, and money – all in order.

Our friends were not able to come and see us off. Bill and Cliff were at work and my 'musketeers' on duty. So at three o'clock we walked out of our room arm in arm, and down the stairs to the waiting taxi. The owners of the house wished us luck and waved until we were out of sight.

When the taxi weaved its way through the maze of the London docks I searched eagerly for the huge liner with the three funnels . . . None to be seen . . . Finally, the taxi stopped outside a forlorn-looking building and deposited us by a group of dejected looking people . . . I caught sight of my liner . . . It was small, grimy and had one funnel! "Oh, *no*," I protested to my husband, "Oh, no, Jimmy, this *can't* be it!"

" 'KASHMIR' ", Jim read out, " 'P. and O.' – this is it all right."

The formalities were brief and soon over, and we all trooped up the gangway onto the greasy deck; we clambered over and around snakes of ropes and coils of wire. And on to the top deck:

Silently we stood against the rail, gazing down into the murky water.

Then Jim put a strong protecting arm around me and said quietly: “You know, my little darling, your mother was quite right . . . You should not have been so emphatic when you were a child . . . you became a nurse, married a doctor, and now you’re on your way to China!”